THERE HAS TO BE
ANOTHER WAY

THERE HAS TO BE
ANOTHER WAY

A doctor's healing journey begins where
medicine ends. The inspiring true story
about the birth of QEC

Dr. Melanie Salmon

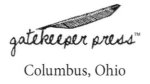

gatekeeper press™

Columbus, Ohio

There Has to Be Another Way: A doctor's healing journey begins where medicine ends. The inspiring true story about the birth of QEC.

Published by Gatekeeper Press
2167 Stringtown Rd, Suite 109
Columbus, OH 43123-2989
www.GatekeeperPress.com

ISBN (paperback): 9781662918599
eISBN: 9781662918605

Cover design: Simon Francis, drawfour.co.za
Copy editor: Biddy Greene
Proofreader: Ethné Clarke
www.qecliving.com

I dedicate this book to all my patients and clients.

Seeing your pain, knowing your suffering,
and hearing about your disappointment in treatments
that were not making a difference,
inspired me to 'find another way'.

Contents

Part 2: The Other Way

Foreword

When I heard that Melanie was writing this book, my immediate response was excitement and "Thank God" – literally. It is an act of courage and profound service for her to be willing to share her story with us.

Over decades, both as a monk and working as a professional coach, I have had the privilege of being with people from all walks of life. Wherever they are from, whatever they share, there's a common theme. It's said in different ways and might be summarised as "I want to be free". Free from the limitations, from the stories, from the past, the heaviness, "the voice in my head". I want to be able to sleep when I'm tired, not ravaged by the endless show-time that's in my mind. I want a healthy pain-free body, clarity, to be content, to be confident, to be able speak up, to know, to discover who I am. I want to be free.

For a long time the word 'trauma' was used only to describe the narrowest of scenarios. It was spoken by those with heads bowed, or with a fiery defiance, and with words aligned to being a survivor. More recently it has become recognised as a word of depth, and it is still often misunderstood.

My own trauma was pushed so far down it wasn't even a thing any more. It was vaulted, neatly labelled: time, place, event, people involved. I knew where all the items were. And I'd "dealt with them". I could describe them. They couldn't touch me anymore. And I could use them to help others understand their journeys.

But my body knew the real score and it kept it. Secretly. Until it couldn't.

I'm a firm believer that when the student is ready, the teacher appears. I'd heard about Melanie through one of my own clients, and my intuition said 'You have to meet her.'

I have worked with leading world experts on shame, vulnerability and transformation. This remarkable woman is the real deal.

Before you turn the page and dive in, let me simply add this.

What you are about to read isn't a story. It's a living experience of a human being. It's written from the heart with a ruthless, bold truth. You'll read about extraordinary circumstances; you might wonder how it was possible for her to keep going. For her even to find the energy to look for another way.

By shining a light so bravely on her own path, Melanie offers you the chance to hear the "me too" within you. Her extraordinary path paves the way for us all – to heal, to be free.

Nic / Mahita Ishaya
Monk, Coach. Co-founder of Remarkable Women
www.remarkablewomen.co.uk

Introduction

This book is my story. It is the story of my personal childhood trauma and how I healed myself from trauma. It is raw and, in places, hard to read. It was hard to write.

The reason that I'm sharing my truth is that I bring a message of hope: it *is* possible to be healed from one's childhood trauma, no matter how bad it was. I have been.

I healed myself completely, using my own unique modality, which I've called 'Quantum Energy Coaching' (QEC). After years spent in Gestalt psychotherapy and other modalities, my deepest core wounds remained out of reach. Gestalt Relational Healing was a necessary and important foundation to address the abandonment and abuse I suffered in childhood, but my essential core wounds remained pivotal in defining who I was and how I functioned in the world.

After several decades practising as a Doctor of Medicine, and years of studying psychotherapy and having psychotherapy, I remained lacking in confidence and with very little feeling of self-worth. I felt disempowered and was easily shamed. I hid behind a mask of professionalism, and drank behind closed doors when the stress became too much.

Despite two mainstream careers, I was frustrated that I was unable to meet the needs of my traumatised patients. My constant lament in those days was: 'There has to be another way!'

Writing prescriptions for drugs felt wrong. Lengthy talk therapy was not within reach of most of my patients. I eventually took early retirement to see if I could develop another way. This book is the story of how I did this.

My wish is that anyone who has suffered the painful disconnection and loneliness arising from childhood trauma will know that there *is* hope, that full healing and connection *is* possible.

Some names have been changed to protect identities.

PART 1

The Journey

CHAPTER 1

Early Childhood

In four weeks' time I will turn seventy. It is 29 December 2017 and I am in South Africa, sitting at my computer looking out onto the garden, watching the slow devastation as the Western Cape drought consumes the plant life. Large brown patches have replaced what was once a lush green lawn surrounding the house. I look beyond to the bay of Somerset West and remember how the sea always made me happy as a child.

Our place of refuge in the summers of early childhood was our annual trip to Umtentweni on the Natal South Coast, where my father's relatives had a small house near the beach. My uncle was the local post office clerk and we stayed with him until, years later, my father invested in an acre of land nearby where we camped each July holiday.

These were happy times for me. My mother did not like camping and usually stayed behind, so our month's holiday was overseen by my young father, who we saw little of at other times. It was magical being with him at the sea, learning to fish, to surf, to explore rock pools. He was always available – for stories and fireside fun and games. These tropical sensory tastes and experiences have been imprinted in my heart and I've spent many years indulging in tropical foods and sensory holiday experiences which capture that 'away from it all' time in Umtentweni.

I look back on my early childhood with mixed feelings. The difficulty for me, in sharing any memories, is the confusing and often overlapping of good experiences and toxic ones. I need to look with courage at those that hurt and damaged me, and I need to honour the experiences that fed and healed me.

I was born in Johannesburg in 1948, to parents who had been married a year. My mother was twenty when I was born; my father twenty-two. My mother had barely left school and, from what I have been able to glean, she had been brought up by reluctant relatives after losing her own mother to alcoholism and her father to far-off Rhodesia, where he worked all his adult life as a doctor. My own father qualified as a lawyer and did his articles in Johannesburg at the same time as Nelson Mandela. It was a time of serious dedication to work in post-war Johannesburg.

My parents had a photographer friend take a portrait of me and my siblings on each birthday. When I was going through psychotherapy in 1989, I came across some of these old photographs. Other than the annual portraits, there seems to be almost no photographic record of my childhood. From these few pictures I was able to see how the look in my eyes changed over successive years. On my second birthday I am full of joy and my eyes are shining and open. I am inviting connection.

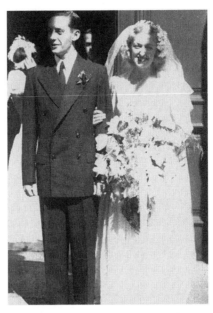

My parents, Edgar and Joan, married in Johannesburg, 1947

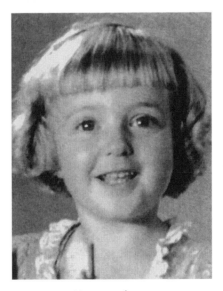

Me, aged two

By the age of three I am more inhibited and watchful. Do I trust the world out there?

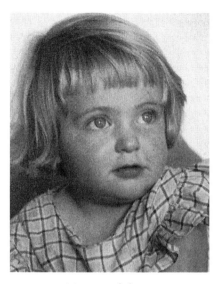

Me, aged three

When I was three, my parents built their own three-bedroomed house in Mondeor, south of Johannesburg. It was a new development surrounded by *koppies*[1], with a river running through it. Mondeor was known as 'the Jewel of the South'. It was set amongst rolling hills, away from the sights and sounds of the city, yet only fifteen minutes' drive from the centre of Johannesburg. I loved this rural village and, as I grew older, I spent much time outdoors, roaming the koppies and

---

[1] A 'koppie' is a small hill.

wandering along the rivers until it was growing dark and I had to return to the house.

Our neighbours were the Bergs, and Susan, the eldest of four daughters, has been my friend ever since. I too was the eldest of four, with two brothers and a sister coming after me. By the time my mother was twenty-seven she had had four children and one miscarriage. She had also recently lost her father and had began drinking heavily.

Today I bought the *Cape Argus* newspaper, with the front page article:

> Enough child killings ... at least 66 children died this year, most of them at the hands of those who knew them ... we will be looking at the root causes of why these children were killed, to start a research project into the killings ... we need to know why our children are being murdered.

I know why children are brutalised. I had a mother who wanted to kill me.

I remember being beaten often, with frequent threats of 'I'll kill you!' Being born to a twenty-year-old, naive, traumatised, disconnected mother, I was emotionally abandoned as well as unpredictably physically brutalised by my mother. By the age of four I had become withdrawn, timid and watchful. A photograph taken on my fourth birthday captures the protective posture of shoulders forwards, head down, cautious gaze. I was already 'frozen'.[2]

I have few memories of early childhood. Many of the details of my narrative come from family stories, usually told by my mother as a source of entertainment. The first story I was told was that breastfeeding me was a deeply shaming experience for her. Apparently a lesbian nurse stood and watched her breastfeed me in the nursing home, passing remarks filled with sexual innuendos during the process. This made my mother feel deeply ashamed of feeding me – and of most other bodily tasks also. By the time I was five years old, I sensed this. It created disgust and disconnection with my own body, resulting in a lifelong self-concept of 'I am disgusting'.

When I was four, my brother Howard was born, and two years later my sister Linda arrived, followed, a year after that, by Clinton. Family pictures show me holding my baby brother in my arms. I remember being called 'Mummy's little helper', a role I adopted to gain attention. When a child does not have their emotional needs met by a responsive, caring parent, they will adapt and shape themselves into whatever they believe they must, to get their attachment needs met. Becoming a helper is one of these.

---

[2] Becoming frozen is an automatic response of 'shut-down' or immobilisation of the autonomic nervous system when trauma is overwhelming.

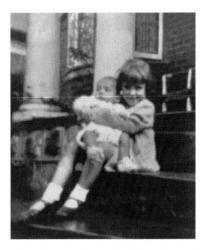

'Mother's little helper', aged four, holding baby brother Howard

My mother was cold, and emotionally distant. She disliked physical contact and pushed me off her lap if I tried to climb up. As a result I soon shut down my desire for physical contact. It has taken me a long time to break down my own distrust and shame in reaching out for support.

My mother was unpredictable and cruel, especially when she drank heavily. She had a tempestuous, jealous relationship with my father who was very often late in coming home from work. Violent verbal abuse regularly led to physical fights between them. I assumed responsibility for protecting the younger children from these alcoholic scenes, while also attempting to protect my mother by intervening in whatever way I could. At the age of six I felt entirely alone, unvalued and full of shame. I was anxious and constantly watchful for signs of danger. The burden of care and protection was weighing heavily on me.

And then at the age of six I was sexually abused.

CHAPTER 2

Being Sexually Abused

I woke up this morning yearning to walk along the Laurensford River in Somerset West. Radloff Park, which is demarcated a safe walking area, runs alongside the river for about three kilometres. I went there this morning and sat for a while on the bank, watching the river flowing over brown, rounded rocks. The sound of the water was exactly what I wanted to hear. I remembered how, as a child, I was able to visit the river in Mondeor whenever I needed to, to sit and watch and listen, as the water washed my soul and spirit clean.

As a child of six, I was allowed out into nature every afternoon to play, returning only when it was suppertime, usually around six o'clock. Then, unexpectedly, the rules changed. My mother had started a secretarial job in Johannesburg and was away during the day. We were left in the care of Dumisani, our young domestic worker, with the instruction that all the children had to rest each afternoon for a couple of hours.

I remember imploring Dumisani to allow me to go outside to play as I had never before spent the afternoon resting. He made a bargain with me: if I rested briefly, with him lying beside me on my bed, he would let me out sooner. For six months, until he was fired for some reason that was never explained to me, I endured almost daily sexual abuse. Dumisani wasn't unkind or frightening. But having to lie beside him on my top bunk-bed, while he ejaculated over my naked body was intensely disgusting to me. Looking back, I can remember feeling detached during the experience and impatient to get outside, to run away as fast as I could afterwards. Our river was several miles from home and it took me at least twenty minutes to reach it. I would run there on my own almost every day, to be beside the flowing water.

Looking back on this experience, my memory is fragmented, brief and without emotion. I am disconnected from these snapshots of happenings, even though the picture is vivid and in colour, and the sounds and smells are powerfully present. To this day I am unable to use a kitchen *lappie* (cloth) as this was what Dumisani used to wipe the semen off my body.

The trauma that I had already suffered at the hands of my mother had made me easy prey for Dumisani's molestation. The sexual abuse lasted only about six months, but it confirmed my already-existing belief that I was disgusting.

On the positive side, I received abundant nurturing from nature. I spent every moment I could playing alone or with my friend Sue from next door, out in the veld or on the koppies, or racing our cork boats along the brown river's rapids. Nature was always a counterpoint to what I missed in human contact. When I climbed the oak tree outside my bedroom window I would sit in its boughs like a child receiving a mother's embrace. In the tree I felt safe, understood, and deeply held. My tree allowed me to recover sufficiently to go back and face each night of terror and uncertainty with my unpredictable and violent mother.

Much later, when I entered Gestalt[3] psychotherapy in my forties, I was frozen emotionally, numbed out and disconnected from authentic feeling. Burnout, while I was working as a GP, was the trigger for my entering therapy.

I began my first therapy session by assuring the therapist that I was merely there for professional reasons: to deal with the stress of my work. I told her that I had had a wonderful and happy childhood and that I was happily married with a mortgage, a good husband and two beautiful sons. I told her that I loved my job as a GP and that I felt guilty for wasting her time. She smiled and said, 'You don't need to have a problem to come for Gestalt therapy.'

My denial did not last long; the following week I began to share with her my childhood history. Thus unfolded the nightmare reality of my childhood and the extent to which

---

[3] Gestalt psychotherapy, developed by Fritz Perls in Johannesburg and the USA in the 1960s, is a client-centred approach to psychotherapy that helps clients focus on the present, and understand what is really happening in their lives right now, rather than what they may perceive to be happening based on past experience.

I had been abused. I began, painfully and slowly, to access memories previously split off from my awareness.

The first memory I shared in therapy was of being aged nine, when my mother told me she had 'a secret to share' that I was to keep strictly to myself. That was the moment my life turned upside down.

CHAPTER 3

Mother's Secret

My early school experiences shaped me deeply, affecting my entire trajectory of learning. Even now, as I write, I notice a low-level anxiety, a slightly sick feeling at the pit of my stomach – a sense of 'it's dangerous to speak out'. I understand why it has taken me so long to begin writing this story.

Mondeor was a small, newly established community. When I was five I attended a make-shift school called The Log Cabin. Classes were held in a small community hall, built with logs and situated in the lowest part of the valley, next to the river. The internal dimensions were large enough to host four classes, Grade 1 to Grade 4, separated from each other by two or three free-standing asbestos dividers. One could hear all the classes in the small space and I imagine it was challenging for teachers to keep children sufficiently quiet while teaching them.

I was excited and positive about going to school. My mother had taught me to read and write before I turned five. According to her, she was bored and had nothing else to do. I was excited to be grown-up enough to walk to school, some twenty minutes away across the veld. I remember the first three weeks vividly. There were about twenty children in my class who were potential playmates and I wanted to excel and make friends as soon as I could.

During lessons I remember being restless and excited, unable to sit still, raising my hand each time the teacher asked a question and jumping up and down to be chosen to answer. After a while, when no one else was answering except me, the teacher asked me to be silent and give the others a turn. This was very hard and confusing as I hoped to shine and be rewarded. After three weeks, the teachers decided to move me to Grade 2 on the basis that I was disruptive and already knew all there was to know of the Grade 1 syllabus.

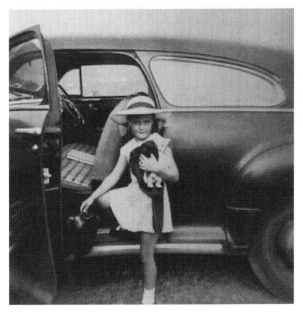

Me, aged five, going to school

I was devastated. And frightened. Suddenly I was with a peer group a year older than me and I was clearly socially out of my depth. I felt punished and lonely. School for me now became unsafe, unpredictable and dangerous. I learned that to shine, to show my cleverness, was not in my best interests. Throughout the rest of my schooldays I suffered from loneliness and a fear of punishment if I dared show what I was capable of. I became a target of bullying. By the time I was nine years old, I was adept at doing well enough academically not to displease my father, and not doing so well that the bullying would escalate. I walked a tightrope, avoiding punishment on both sides of the line.

What I am struck by as I write about these traumatic events and remember the loneliness, the uncertainty and the ever-present danger, is how robust and resilient I remained. I remember playing happily with my trusted friend Sue from next door. I loved making 'houses' with her. I built houses endlessly and obsessively, from tree houses to tiny villages in the sandpit. Through play I was able to create safety and happiness within the house that I inhabited in my imagination.

In spite of all the traumas and challenges I endured, I was relatively happy and carefree. I had a distant relationship with my mother and when my father was around, was able to enjoy his company by playing cricket and other 'tomboy' sports. And then one day, things changed.

It was a lovely sunny Sunday afternoon at the start of spring in 1957. My aunt Maureen and my uncle Arthur, with my younger cousins Carol and Kevin, were visiting us for a braai[4]. My uncle and aunt were both doctors; they lived and worked in the north of Johannesburg. My uncle always brought us comics and chocolates. I loved seeing them and really appreciated their visiting us. I remember taking my comic and quietly moving off to lie in the make-shift house that I'd built earlier at the end of the grapevine. I wanted to read in peace, undisturbed by the younger ones playing in the orchard. The sun was just setting and it was getting slightly dark.

And then I heard my mother calling from the back door for me to come inside. She had to call twice. I was deeply absorbed in my comic book, the superhero tales of Batman and Robin. I jumped up and made for the kitchen door. The adults were sitting around the outside fire, and I could hear the voices of the other children playing in the orchard beyond.

I stepped inside, calling to my mother, 'Here I am. Where are you?'

The entire house was in darkness. I heard my mother calling from the lounge and walked quickly through the dining room. I was unable to see her clearly in the darkness of the lounge beyond the table and chairs, and when I reached up to put on the light she shouted, 'Don't switch the light on! Come here… I want to talk to you.'

I stood dead still. My heart seemed to stop in that moment. I could only make out my mother's silhouette against the far window. I felt instantly afraid.

---

[4] A 'braai' (pronounced 'bry') is a barbeque.

'I have something to tell you,' she said, 'and I want you to promise me that you will never, under any condition whatsoever, tell this to anyone!'

I remained silent, frozen to the spot, unable to speak, unable to breathe with the tension of what was to come...

'You know that I've been seeing the doctors recently and having blood tests... Well, I had the results yesterday. They told me I have leukaemia. That's cancer of the blood. They say I have only twelve months to live.'

I was dumbstruck; unable to move. I couldn't grasp what this meant. I heard the words 'only twelve months to live' and realised that this meant I would be losing my mother. I was hearing something so big, so frightening... It threatened my own survival.

'You are not to tell anyone; not ever. This is just between us,' she finished.

Her last words rang in my ears as I walked woodenly out of the back door and into the darkness of the descending night. In that moment my life changed completely.

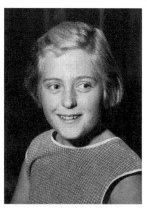

Me, aged nine, 1957

CHAPTER 4

The Secret Divorce

I have had a troubled day today. I went walking again along the Laurensford River. I have been feeling vulnerable and emotional. I woke up after an unpleasant dream, which is unusual for me these days. I've had an ache around my chest and upper back, as if my heart was breaking. At times I felt quite faint and wanted to vomit. I lay down until it passed.

Writing my story, the last part especially, has triggered a physical and emotional response that is new to me. In the telling of the story in therapy I was in a detached head space, clear, practical, and sensible. Today I am distraught. I am also outraged, grief-stricken and nauseous. It is incomprehensible to me that I agreed to what was in effect a sentence of imprisonment.

To ask a child to hold the knowledge of the impending death of her mother without being able to seek support, and to keep it a secret from everyone, is unbelievably cruel. I am shocked and appalled. I fully understand how this single event shaped my entire life and why it became my life's mission to find a way to heal the core wo unds of childhood. I understand why I became a doctor.

It is a day since I wrote that. I am recovered and have been enjoying the post-Christmas sunshine while lying at the pool. As I was pondering my love of sunshine, a passion ever since I can remember, my mind drifted to a sunny holiday when I was nine years old, before my life came to a standstill.

We had gone in July as a family, invited by Portuguese clients of my father, for a holiday in Lourenço Marques, in Mozambique. We stayed in a beach rondavel[5], only yards from the warm Indian Ocean. It was magical and different from our Natal summer holidays: hotter, exotic, full of new sights and smells and adventures. My father's client, George, was the owner of a large photographic business and a retail outlet. He was very wealthy and entertained us lavishly, giving all four of us children huge presents from his toy shop in the city. The beautiful doll I received, I kept for years in my cupboard. In a box. I would never play with it. Playing was lost to me through my ever-present state of trauma.

Most evenings we dined at exotic coastal restaurants, where I learned to eat prawns and mussels fresh from the sea. George and his brother owned a speedboat and taught us to waterski. It was a heady and abundant experience, and for the first time we children were not excluded from the long evening

---

[5] A circular 'African' dwelling with a conical thatched roof.

meals that stretched late into the night. I understand now why I am drawn to Mediterranean countries, and why I invested in a property by the sea in northern Spain, spending summer holidays there during my two decades of living in England.

But something troubling happened on that Mozambique holiday. As usual, my father had taken us all out to swim in the safe sea pool in front of the main restaurant and marina. My mother didn't enjoy swimming and stayed back, sitting under an umbrella at the tea room. We were far out to sea with our father, having fun and shouting to each other as we played. I could see my mother in the distance, having her tea and reading something. Suddenly my father shouted at us to get out, to swim to the shore, as he himself swam ahead alarmingly quickly. I helped the younger ones get back to shore while watching my father run up the beach and into the tearoom. I saw him grab something from my mother's hand; it looked like a letter and I watched as they struggled violently at the table. He was shouting and very angry.

We were never told what had happened, nor why my parents were so angry with each other. We had to stay in our beach bungalow, and look after ourselves, for the remaining few days. It was awful. There was a bad atmosphere and the holiday seemed to be over. We did not see 'Uncle George' ever again.

At the age of nine I was unable to make sense of the signals and behaviour of my parents. Secrets abounded. It was only when I turned eighteen and required my father's legal permission for something, that I learned from my mother that they had divorced that year – soon after the Mozambique trip and a few weeks before my mother told me that she had terminal cancer.

My father, a divorce lawyer himself, did not want the scandal of his own divorce to impact his business. My parents managed to arrange their divorce secretly, without anyone in the family or among their circle of friends knowing. My father obtained legal custody of all four children and 'allowed' my mother to stay on at home to care for us, provided she 'did not put a foot wrong', referring – I discovered later – to her frequent affairs. He made no attempt though, to curtail her increasing consumption of alcohol.

The agreement apparently was that they would continue 'living as before', as husband and wife, being present together for family celebrations such as birthdays and Christmas. We saw significantly less of my father from 1957 onwards – just at the time when I needed him to help with my dying mother. I had no context for the estranged behaviour of my father and his absence, and I felt abandoned, frightened and lost.

I have only vague memories of the years that followed. I turned eleven when I entered my last year of primary school, Standard 5. I was chosen to be a prefect and received a special prefect's blazer. I had grown accustomed to school and was an active participant in sports. My mother's illness absorbed all my focus and attention. I dropped out of netball and the athletics team, and my schoolwork began to decline. The headmaster, our Standard 5 class teacher, sent reports home stating, 'Melanie is no longer applying herself'. Oddly enough, the reason for this was never investigated – in those days there was no understanding that a child's sudden underachievement might be linked to trouble at home.

I was withdrawn and miserable at school and rapidly again became the target of bullying. All of this did not touch me much. Looking back even now I can feel how indifferent I was to criticism and attack. My only concern, day and night, was how my mother was doing. Often I would feel the onset of panic during a lesson, thinking, 'Maybe today is the day she will die!'

Sometimes I would slip out in the middle of class, and walk several kilometres home, to check on her. Her response was always a casual 'What are you doing here?' I assured her I was just checking to see if she was alright. She happily accepted my truanting and did nothing to communicate with the school in my defence. I did this so frequently, and without satisfactory explanation, that the school took away my prefect's blazer. It was deeply shaming.

That year was the loneliest and most terrifying of my life. I had trouble sleeping and was disturbed by nightmares of my mother dying. I would wake up and tiptoe into her bedroom and stand next to her bed to check that she was still breathing. If I could see her chest moving, I knew she was alive and I could go back to bed. My mother spent much time in bed. She drank very heavily each evening, sometimes to the point of vomiting and collapsing over the toilet. Regularly I would have to clean up the alcohol-infused vomit and get her to bed. I remember the inner struggle between pulling back in disgust and reaching out compassionately to help my dying mother.

On the few evenings that my father came home early, there would be horrible drunken fights between them. I was now extremely worried about my mother's condition, so I would listen through the door until their voices were raised to the point of physical attack, then open the door and run into the room to protect her, putting myself physically between them. Often I received vicious blows, but I felt nothing. What mattered to me was that she was being protected. I also protected the younger ones from the impact of these frightening experiences. I remember often herding them out of the nearby bedroom and into the living room, where less could be heard. I would tell them stories and play games with them with one ear on the background sounds, making sure that I didn't need to return to the battlefield. Both parents seemed oblivious to any of our needs as small children.

During that year I was given the additional task of washing and ironing for the family. Most days I spent hours after school in the laundry out at the back, using the old-fashioned washing machine with a mangle, then hanging the clothes up on the outside line. It was tiring but satisfying work and I would have enjoyed this solitary task if I had not been expected to babysit my younger siblings at the same time. I became very good at multi-tasking.

A typical school day for me started at 4.30 a.m. While everyone was asleep I was able to do school work for a couple of hours. I have always loved the dawn with its gentle light and bird calls, offering hope to each new day. Throughout my life I have treasured early mornings, a time quiet enough to work undisturbed. I am even writing this story at 5.30 a.m.

By 7 a.m. I was supervising the others as they washed and dressed for school. I made sure that Mother was still alive, and took her a tray of tea in bed. I made breakfast for all of us. By then we had a permanent 'house boy' called Isaac, who did the major heavy work in the house and garden, but I still had to do the meals and laundry. I walked to school with my brother Howard, who was then six years old. I can't remember what the arrangements for the little ones were.

Aside from sporadic bullying, I was generally left alone at school. School work was easy enough, in all my subjects. As long as I kept attention away from myself I could blend unnoticed into the background. I remember liking all subjects equally, apart one which stands out in my memory: Art. In Mrs Pincus' art class we were given creative sculpture to do. The first project was to sculpt something out of Sunlight soap. I was totally absorbed. I can still smell the soap and feel its slippery green surface. I sculpted a skyscraper. I was very good. But this drew attention to myself, so I backed off. Sunlight soap is still sold in South Africa today; my husband uses it, and when I catch the smell I return immediately to Mrs Pincus' class, holding that completed skyscraper, feeling caught between the excitement of being creative and the fear of bullying.

After school I walked home with Howard. South African primary schools closed at 1 p.m. for the younger classes and

24

at 2 p.m. for the older children. Howard had to wait for me until I was ready to go home at 2 as Mother was ill and still mostly in bed and could not fetch him by car. It's a long way to walk for such a small child and I used to stop at the shops on the way home to buy him a lollipop with money I stole from my father's 'sixpence tin' in which he saved small change. We were not given pocket money or sweets and this was a risky act on my part. I felt protective of Howard and desperately upset that I couldn't stop him from having beatings. He regularly got into trouble. He wasn't as fast a learner as I was and seemed to upset my parents and his teachers very easily. I remember once walking him home after a caning he had received at school. He was silent and white-faced all the way. My treat helped us both a little.

My father came home less and less often, and my mother spent more and more time in bed. He gave the excuse of being 'too busy', saying he had to work hard as 'money doesn't grow on trees!' That year he changed towards me and was much stricter and more irritable when I asked for help with homework. I became reluctant to show him anything as his attitude was always that it 'wasn't good enough'. My mother was totally indifferent to my school work and so I kept trying harder to please my father. At least he took an interest. But I missed the fun times we had had, and the laughter. Our home had become very gloomy and dark.

I missed my play times, too, with Sue next door. Previously in the holidays we would go out for hours into the koppies, alone or with the younger ones. But now I felt I couldn't risk being too far away from Mother. She needed me to wait on her in bed, with trays of tea, lunch and so on. I got very anxious if I wasn't within calling distance of her. I kept telling myself 'this might be the day she dies; then you'll be sorry'. I settled for making a hole in the hedge between Sue's back garden and ours and we would sit there talking through the hedge. We no longer made houses.

Towards the end of that year my father came home increasingly rarely. When he did, he encouraged me to take an interest in playing tennis. He said he now belonged to a tennis club in Johannesburg and I could come along on Sundays and he would teach me to play. I jumped at the chance of being with him again, away from the house. I was concerned about leaving Mother for a whole afternoon, but by that time she seemed to be improving; she was spending less time in bed. I accepted my father's invitation and went to his club at the Cottesloe Mine Hospital in Johannesburg one Sunday afternoon. There he introduced me to his new girlfriend, a nurse called Chrystelle. I was extremely embarrassed and upset. How could he betray my poor, dying mother? I struggled with loyalty to her but in the end I gave in to the need to be with my father, under any circumstances. But I was not happy at having to choose between them.

The solution for me was resolved in eating.

One afternoon after tennis, cakes were left over and Chrystelle gave me a granadilla-icing cake to take home to the family. I kept it secretly in my bedroom cupboard, eating under the covers after everyone had gone to bed. I discovered how much better I felt, how much easier it was to fall asleep if my tummy was full. Thereafter, every night, I took several thick slices of bread and jam to bed. Thus began my addiction to sugar.

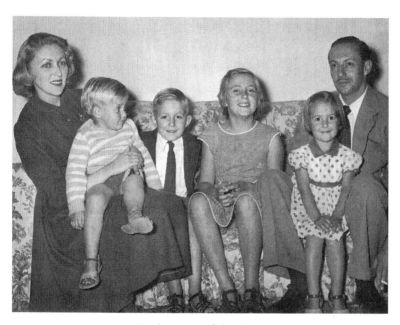

1957, the year of the divorce

CHAPTER 5

High School Years

In 1960 I moved to high school. Sir John Adamson High School was brand new. It was built at the top of the range of hills overlooking Mondeor and drew (white) children from all over the southern suburbs of Johannesburg. A brick double-storey building, it was imposing and beautiful, with distant views over the hills of the south. The playgrounds were dusty and there were no sports facilities yet, but to me my new school was lovely. We wore navy blue and green uniforms with white shirts and ties. I felt very grown up.

During my first year, the classes only went up to Form Three (Standard 8/Grade 10), as there weren't enough senior pupils for the final two years. Once again I grew with the school. There were several hundred children at the school the year it opened, and each year was divided academically into four streams or classes. I was in the A class with about thirty others. I knew only a few children in my class and felt relaxed and pleased about this. I was already an expert at walking the line between doing well enough yet not standing out and attracting attention. I had no interest in making friends and I enjoyed the anonymity.

Looking after Mother and the younger ones continued to dominate my world, and high school was simply a brief respite from this bigger duty. Yet slowly things began to change. I noticed Mother was looking better and becoming less in need of me. When she had not died in the twelve months she had originally suggested, I accepted this as some sort of divine good luck. I nevertheless remained silent as requested, and did not question her improved health. I was as assiduous as ever, watching for any signs of her impending demise. She regularly had physical 'bad turns', as she called them, with palpitations and the feeling that she was about to die. Uncle Arthur would come out on these occasions and do a full medical examination, assuring me that everything was 'fine'.

On one of these occasions I was very close to telling him my 'secret'. I ran after him as he was leaving, saying I had something to tell him. He got out of the car and said, 'Yes, what is it?'

I was tongue-tied. I simply could not say anything. 'Nothing,' I mumbled, and turned miserably away.

That year I entered puberty. I started menstruating and was shocked when, during class one day, I found blood on my underwear. My mother had not prepared me for this. I remember feeling deeply ashamed when I told her after school, and shared her embarrassment in having to buy me sanitary towels. We were both disgusted by my body and its discharges. Soon after, she told me we had to go shopping for 'a brassiere' as I was 'developing'. Again I was mortified and managed to put this off for months.

I was a tomboy and loved climbing trees and playing cricket and there was no way I could embrace any idea of femininity. Instead I threw myself into learning to play tennis. As I've mentioned, my father took a special interest in my tennis. He paid for lessons with an ex-Wimbledon coach, telling me that one day I would be able to represent South Africa at Wimbledon. He decided that, to facilitate this outcome, we needed to have our own tennis court, so that I could practise every day. Over the weekends he and Isaac built a clay court on land that had been purchased behind our home to have a house built for my paternal grandparents.

By the time I was thirteen the clay tennis court had been completed and, with it, a large cement wall to practise against. I was excited. My father and I were sharing a lot of time together and I eagerly agreed to using my dawn waking each day to be on the court, practising against the wall. He was still sleeping at home and would join me around 6 a.m. to give me instruction. I soon discovered that this wasn't a good idea. His quick temper and impatience rapidly created in me an experience bordering on panic. The more he shouted, the more I missed. I came to dread the early mornings and the tennis lessons with him, but I was far too afraid to show any negative reaction.

I played tennis for two years and was chosen to play to in the school team. My coach entered me into the Transvaal Regional Tennis Championships for under 14s at Ellis Park,

Johannesburg. My father was bursting with pride. He boasted about me to all his friends, and when I was with him, he would introduce me as 'the child who would one day be a tennis star'. It was excruciating. I came to hate tennis.

I did enter the championships though, and reached the Under 14s final round. Then came a moment which changed my tennis career. I was 2–0 up in the third set of the finals when I saw my father arrive with a whole group of friends from the tennis club. They sat down in the stands to watch. Something inside me snapped. I had had enough. I decided that my only way out was to lose. I lost the game and set spectacularly. My father and his friends came rushing up afterwards to see what had happened. I remained silent, looking at the ground. They told themselves that I must be ill.

I never did get to Wimbledon. I stopped lessons and withdrew from the school team. I told my father that, as I was entering Standard 8 the next year, I wanted to put all my time and energy into my studies. It was a clever move. I knew he prized academic achievement above all else, so he left me alone. He took for granted that I did not need coaching for school work and I saw very little of him after this. It was a bittersweet victory.

That July we had a holiday in Margate. Margate is only three miles from Umtentweni and this time my mother came along because we were to stay in a hotel and not camp on the plot. I was thrilled. We hadn't been on holiday with my father for three years and I felt excited and full of anticipation. It was a tense time though as my parents remained distant and argumentative. My father taught me to surf on an inflatable bodyboard and I spent hours every day out on the waves.

It was on this holiday, just as I had begun to enjoy moments of being carefree and confident, that my father told me something that would alter my self-image for the rest of my life.

On the beach one day, while I was enjoying an ice-cream he looked at me and exclaimed, 'You're getting too fat! You'll have to lose some weight before any man will look at you.'

I was devastated. I had been unaware of my body or how others saw me. I knew I was disgusting on the inside – and now I was also disgusting on the outside.

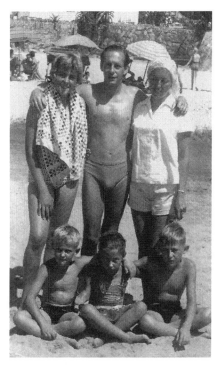

'You're getting too fat!' The family on Margate beach, 1960

CHAPTER 6

A Teenage Confidante

I felt trapped in an ever-smaller box. My mother, her health improving over the months, was nevertheless very dependent on me. She used me as her emotional confidante. She needed all my attention and had a not-so-subtle way of getting me to cancel any outings or parties or other events, to remain at her side. She would become 'sick' just before I was about to go out. Each time I told myself, 'Stay with her, in case this is the day she dies.' I didn't even get to go to my Matric farewell. I was too consumed with caring and responsibility to see or understand how I was being manipulated. Instead I believed myself privileged to share her adult concerns about my wayward father. Also I felt pleased that I was finally having a relationship with her. It helped my loneliness. Not being with my peer group seemed a small sacrifice and, besides, my father had convinced me that I was ugly and unattractive.

My mother had recovered sufficiently in my high school years to take on the production of the annual high school concert. She did this three years running. I found myself in the midst of a whole new atmosphere, a scene of creativity and fun hitherto unknown to me. My mother had trained as an actor and dancer before she got married. She produced brilliant musicals at Sir John High School. I always got a small part, but shyness prevented me from doing more. I loved those productions and considered my life to be quite magical. As long as I did not stray away from Mother's side, and did exactly as she asked, all was good. Our close relationship was totally confluent and absorbing.

Throughout my school life I did not have any really close friends – my mother was my life, and everything else paled into insignificance beside her. I remained her protector and carer, developing an unusual ability to detect anything amiss. Twice during my high school years she was admitted to the Johannesburg General Hospital for abdominal surgery. I remember catching three buses from Mondeor to the hospital to visit her every afternoon after school, and take her clean nighties.

My father stayed away more as I grew older. It was a relief not to have to deal with the fights at night and I accepted that he was no longer part of our lives. Mother's heavy drinking continued unabated. She drank every night, to the point of passing out. By 8 p.m. she was usually unconscious. This did mean, however, that I was able to study at night after the younger ones had been fed and put to bed.

I was developing a routine that I could manage. By now I was committed to studying and doing well enough to go to university. I had less flak now in the A-stream class as there were others who were better than me. This allowed me freedom to do well in exams. I remember the moment, in Standard 8, when Lynette Ward joined our class. She had come from Durban. After the first end-of-term tests she showed herself to be brilliant at Maths, far better than me. I was delighted. I made friends with her immediately, even though she was as shy and as withdrawn as I was. I felt I had an ally.

Aside from her drinking, Mother was no longer taking to bed. After that first confession of 'terminal cancer', she never mentioned any health issues again. Nor did I, as this remained my honour-bound secret, not for discussion, ever. She seemed happier too, and more settled. Our annual July trips to the sea with my father had stopped. My mother replaced this with her own holiday, hiking in the Drakensberg mountains in Natal. This is the most splendid mountain range I have ever known. Mountains fed my soul, and to this day I surround myself with mountains. As I look out my window right now, I see the Hottentots-Holland range of mountains of Somerset West, beyond the razor wire.

When I see old photographs of my young mother out in nature, I understand why I believed I was the luckiest person in the world to have such a wonderful mother. I would do anything for her, give up anything instantly for her. I loved her with my whole heart and wanted to treasure every single moment we shared. I knew she was vulnerable and could die any day, and I got to treasure the good times and make little of the bad times.

I was less effusive about my father, who remained mostly absent in our lives. When I saw him he was almost always critical and judgemental. After my having disappointed him at tennis, he left me alone for a couple of years, but as Matric approached, he again put pressure on my academic work. He suggested that I should follow in the footsteps of his sister, my aunt, Maureen Salmon. Maureen had received the high accolade of the 'Woman of the Year' award for her exceptional role in running the Johannesburg General Hospital. My father decided that medicine would be a fitting career for me.

My mother converted to Catholicism when I was fourteen. She had been giving elocution lessons to some of the priests and brothers at a Salesian Catholic boys' school. Since I went everywhere with her, I was also exposed to their friendliness and kindness. It was natural to want to become a Catholic and I too converted to Catholicism, when I turned eighteen.

At fifteen, I suffered an embarrassing and confusing dilemma, one which I could not resolve. I was convinced I was actually a boy ... that there must have been a terrible mistake and that my mother was dressing me up in girl's clothing. On the inside I felt masculine: strong, capable, responsible. I had no feminine feelings, as I understood them to be. I had never played with dolls, I disliked and mistrusted girls and I hated wearing dresses. I still played tennis, rode horses and climbed trees. My best time alone, if I could slip away, was still to be in the veld, making bush houses in the koppies, cutting away scrubby branches with my penknife.

Of course I did not share any of this, and instead channelled my growing fear into religion. I went to Mass almost daily, and prayed that God would deliver me from this burden of confusion. Study was becoming stressful, and to de-stress I would attend an occasional weekend silent retreat, on my own, at a small Catholic retreat centre. I loved being alone there; having the space to myself.

On one of these weekends, I was so burdened with the dilemma of being a boy in female clothes that I decided to confess this openly to the retreat master, a young good-looking priest. I made an appointment with him and with tremendous difficulty, told him my worst fear.

I can still see his earnest face across the desk from me. He said, 'You are the most feminine young woman I have ever met! If you were my daughter, I would be proud of you!'

I was so relieved that I actually cried. I remember him passing me his handkerchief. I never again doubted my gender.

CHAPTER 7

A New Reality: Denial

It is difficult to stay present on this 15th day of January 2018, here in Somerset West. The light over the mountains is slightly pink and they stand out clear and defined against the pale blue sky. A row of tall blue gums lines the far end of the property. I can't shake what feels like depression. I'm immersed in my teenage life to the extent that I am that fifteen year old again, waiting to turn sixteen in the January when I enter my final year of school.

I feel an inexplicable heaviness around beginning to write about my Matric year, which is strange as my sixteenth year was, in memory, the best school year of all. It was the only year I kept a personal diary. I bought a hard-covered exercise book and labelled it 'My Diary'. I kept this diary over the years, along with a handful of photographs, the only evidence of my childhood. Those pictures are here in this story.

When I was forty and early on in my therapy, I took my diary to Freda, my therapist, believing that if I read from the book, she would have an accurate account of what my life at home had really been like. I was becoming confused in therapy as the return of memories began to play out a story totally different from my original claim that 'I had a perfectly happy childhood'. I needed to prove that this was so and I decided that Freda and I would have to read through this diary, a first-hand witness account of my sixteenth year.

But something very odd happened. As I began to read out loud to Freda from my diary, I saw that, at sixteen, I had entered a state of absolute denial. Freud would call this 'repression'. I described both my parents in terms that I knew were impossible. I spoke of my mother as 'warm and loving' and my father as 'not a devil' but 'a hard-working man who needed my compassion and understanding'. I vowed, 'with God's help' (by now I was very religious) to 'work harder at helping them both'. I gave thanks to God 'for my blessings in having such a wonderful family'. Page after page for a full year, the projection of 'wonderful, beautiful, kind and loving' was put onto what in actuality was cold, harsh, selfish and manipulative from my mother, and punitive criticism and pressure from my father.

I was shocked. I stared at what I had written and did not know what to do with this contradiction. I was deeply confused, frightened. I felt ashamed. I assumed I was a liar of the very worst kind. Later on, and even in my Gestalt training, I learned about the concept of cognitive dissonance. This is the brain's response when faced suddenly with two opposing points of view. It is very disturbing to say the least. When it happened to me I struggled enormously with self-trust and a fractured self-image.

In my matric year I saw what was in front of me as life-giving, loving and healthy. In reality I was immersed in a worsening situation. My mother's alcoholic behaviour had escalated and she had become reckless. Several times I saw her having sex on the sofa in the evenings with men she picked up casually. It was getting extremely hard to juggle my responsibilities and protect my younger siblings from what I believed was disgusting and dangerous for them to know about. And on top of it all I was entering a year of serious and committed study.

The relationship with my mother by then was totally schizophrenic. Or bipolar. She was two entirely different people, changing each day from morning to evening. In the mornings she would wake up cheerful and interested in me, often treating the family to a breakfast of her special scones. Whatever had happened the night before was forgotten. I remember after watching her having sex on the sofa, looking into her eyes the next day for guilt or even some shame – and there was nothing. Nothing.

Occasionally we would visit the Garden Centre before school to buy plants for her gardening projects. I see now where I got my deep love of gardening from. They were magical moments in those wonderful South African garden centres, filled with brilliant colour and fresh morning smells. Each day I set off to school, hopeful that my mother would stay as she was in the mornings.

By late afternoon, after my studies, Mother was already changing. She would actually make our supper, because I had to study in the late afternoons. By five she was drinking whisky, and by six, before supper was ready, the kitchen was a disaster area. Her drunkenness was concerning. It wasn't safe for her to be working at a hot stove, but she became nasty and lashed out if I commented or tried to help. Her personality altered totally under the influence of alcohol. She became aggressive, loud-mouthed and swore often. Our meals were badly prepared and often undercooked or overcooked. We quietly and quickly ate what was prepared and got out of the kitchen as fast as we could, leaving mother to finish her alcohol and stagger to bed; she was often asleep by seven thirty.

My relationship with my mother was unpredictable and kept me constantly anxious as I didn't know who I was going to be with at any given time. I had to meet her where she was – to accept being 'loved' in the morning in a needy and manipulative way, and in the evenings being rejected and sworn at. I also had to face a dramatic swing from being put on a pedestal with praise and accolades, which felt false, to being relegated to a gutter existence and being described as 'a slut and a whore'. There was no middle ground.

Our three-bedroomed small bungalow was noisy, disruptive and difficult to study in. Already I was up at dawn studying before the others awoke, but I also needed time to study after the evening meal. My father asked my grandparents if I could move in with them. By this time they were living behind us in the adjoining property and had a spare room.

They agreed, and each evening I would leave after the chores were done and walk over to their house, where I would study and sleep over. Howard was now old enough to look after the younger children

Sadly – despite having offered me a quiet workplace – my grandparents were hostile and distant and did not really welcome my presence. My grandmother in particular always had a sour face. Later, when I was studying medicine, I learned that Parkinson's diseases can paralyse the muscles of the face, creating a permanent 'mask'. She had a permanent scowl and she did have Parkinson's, but I wasn't aware of this at that stage. I was uncomfortable being in the house, yet relieved at the same time and grateful for the absolute quiet it afforded. I worked in their spare bedroom, which was a green room with a green candlewick bedspread. I loved the order and cleanliness, which contrasted with my own bedroom at home – shared with my sister and always busy and full and noisy. I would sit at the tiny table in the room and study until ten. My grandad would wake me at five with a cup of coffee made from their old-fashioned coffee percolator machine. I can still hear the bubbling it made as it percolated on the stove and taste the horribly weak coffee, which I found distasteful but dared not mention. I remember being glad each day to leave hurriedly and go home, yet dreading what I might find there.

I have been thinking a lot about my sixteenth year and about how writing this part of my story is different, harder. I think it's the confusion and discomfort I feel when sharing how I repressed the truth. This distorted perception, recorded in my diary, of 'perfect happiness' was so complete that it remained unquestioned for the next twenty-four years.

However I did experience good times that year, times when I was away from Mother and the chaotic household. I spent the July holiday in Umtentweni, camping with my father and two of his good friends – a happy married couple with two well-balanced daughters, slightly younger than me. My best friend Sue and her family also holidayed at Southbroom, near to us, and we would all met on Margate beach. The highlight was to attend the dances on Saturday nights at the Palm Grove Hotel. It was the early sixties and the Beatles music had just reached South Africa. I danced my socks off at the Palm Grove every Saturday night. I never wanted to leave Margate.

I enjoyed my matric year. I was a prefect once more, and this time I kept my lovely navy blue prefect blazer. We had a prefects' room, and at break-times we would play music on a record player. I hung out with a small group of girls and I was able to have fun while keeping my distance. I had many male companions, and throughout medical school these easy friendships helped me to feel supported while avoiding intimacy. I loved my school subjects, particularly English and Art. Art classes allowed me an expression previously shut down on, and soon I was certain that at university I would study for a BA and do English and Art.

I was about to apply to the University of the Witwatersrand ('Wits') in Johannesburg to do a BA when my father objected.

He talked to his sister, my Aunt Maureen, and suddenly I found myself being visited by Maureen's friend, a well known professor from the Wits Medical School. My parents informed me that Prof Gear was here to 'talk sense into me' and they left the two of us alone in the lounge. I was dismayed and dumbstruck. I looked across at this very tall man in his grey suit and tie, and waited in embarrassed silence. He proceeded to ask me in a very formal way, why I wanted to do a BA. I told him I loved English and Art and that I wanted to be a journalist.

'What do you know at your age, sixteen?' he responded. 'What can you write about?' He went on, ' If you do medicine, you will be twenty-two when you qualify. You will have more experience of life. You'll have something to write about then. I suggest you do medicine!'

And that is how I agreed to go to medical school. His argument made sense. But the real factor for me was my instinctive 'obedience to authority'. I had no experience of arguing with my elders. I had no idea what I truly wanted. I was totally conditioned to follow orders and to expect that others knew what was best for me and my life. So once more I sublimated my artistic creative desires and accepted that I had to follow in my aunt's footsteps. 'Besides,' my father told me, 'she is paying half your university fees.' I was to be absolutely grateful for this help, he said, and I had to work hard to prove I was worthy of it.

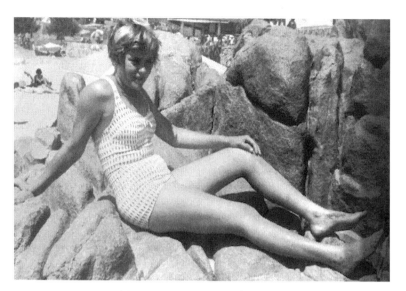

Me, at Margate, aged sixteen

CHAPTER 8

Entering Medical School

As I look at the photograph of my sixteen-year-old self on the rocks at the seaside, it's difficult to imagine anyone allowing such a young, naive, insecure and frozen child into medical school with a hundred and ten students, some of whom were already young men. White South African boys had to do two years of army service, and many elected to do this straight after school and so were nineteen years and older in first year of Medicine. I was totally out of my depth in this new environment. It was a culture shock: I came from the wrong side of town, the south, and the rich and educated people came from the north. My accent was wrong, and for the first year I was afraid to speak for fear that people would spot my 'southern suburbs' accent.

I was desperately lost and lonely at university. First year medical students did four subjects: Botany, Zoology, Physics and Chemistry. The lectures were, it seemed to me, in a foreign language, and no assistance from lecturers was available at all. I was terrified of everything. I felt stupid and hopelessly incapable and I was too afraid to admit this to anyone. I decided to seek refuge in 'God's House'. I discovered a small Catholic chapel on a corner below the university. I managed to attend Mass there every single day at 6 a.m. before my classes started. I prayed in desperation for help to get me through. I did not believe I had either the intelligence or the stamina to endure this course.

What was particularly distressing was the laboratory work, the 'practicums' in Zoology. We had to kill the brains of live frogs and dissect them before the heart stopped beating. 'Pithing frogs' was done by sticking a long needle through the back of the brain behind the eyes, into the skull cavity and wiggling the needle about until the frog was 'brain dead' although its muscles still worked. You knew it was brain dead when it emitted a haze of white sweat all over its skin which gave out an unpleasant odour. Just writing this now is bringing tears to my eyes. I have to stop.

I've been sitting in the fading light of this summer day next to my fish pond. We have several bull frogs there, now singing in chorus as the sun sets. I apologised to them all on behalf of humanity for killing frogs in order to learn about science. I am ashamed of the human race.

That year was a living nightmare. I cried each evening, begging my mother to allow me to leave medical school. To no avail. My father had the power over this decision and I dared not approach him. He began building a 'study rondavel' for me in our back yard, clearing away the orchard. Together with Isaac he made concrete bricks and within six months they had built a large rondavel. It was for me, the medical student, to have my own place to study, undisturbed. Now there was definitely no chance of leaving my course.

In my second year, we moved away from the main university campus and up the hill to the Medical School itself, situated in Hillbrow, behind Johannesburg General Hospital. I had begun to adjust to the routine of lectures and self-directed learning. Second year medicine consisted of only two subjects, Anatomy and Physiology. I was almost looking forward to subjects that felt more like medicine and less like science. But I had a further shock in store: the study of anatomy and the dissection practicums.

Each day, for half a day, five days a week, we had to dissect the human cadaver. My first sight came without any forewarning or preparation. On that first day we chatted happily on the way to the nearby dissection hall and on entering were divided into groups of six per body. I looked out at the hall, and saw row upon row of dead bodies under white plastic sheets. A whole hall of dead people. The students continued laughing and chatting as they took up their places on stools, six to an anatomy table with a junior assistant allocated to each group. Then the cloth was removed and the smell hit me. Formalin. The body in front of me was of a white female, old, yellow, skinny, wizened, eyes sunken into the skull. I looked on in shock. I couldn't move or speak. I had never seen a dead body before. The men at my table laughed and joked, finding my fear and revulsion amusing. I hated Anatomy and was appalled at the smell of formalin. I can still smell it. It remained in my nose and mouth the entire year, affecting everything I ate.

What was equally shocking for me as time went on, was the callous attitude cultivated by some students towards the bodies they dissected, the cadavers being a source of humour. On one occasion I joined my group to find them playing with a length of intestine from our cadaver's body, swinging it around, hitting each other in fun. Students often brought their sandwiches and stayed to eat their lunch around the cadaver if they hadn't finished the week's assignment. It made me feel sick.

I was 'frozen', in the neurological sense of the word, because of my childhood trauma. This made me emotionally detached and disconnected from myself and others. I operated only from my head and remained numbed out from the neck down. As a result of the exposure to shocking experiences throughout medical training, my peers were becoming desensitised, a process of closing down one's feelings, which resulted in callous and indifferent behaviour. I did not escape desensitisation myself, and, by the time I reached my house-officer years working in Casualty, I too had achieved a black sense of humour that deflected the gory horrors that we had to deal with every night.

Finally third year arrived, and with it the promise of proper medical subjects. At last we would be learning about illness through the subjects of Pathology, Haematology and Pharmaceuticals. I had reasoned that my medical career would be my one great opportunity to discover how I could better help my mother with her terminal illness.

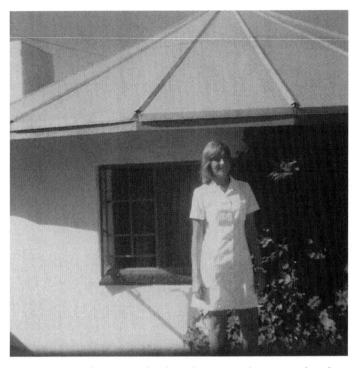

Me, second year medical student, outside my rondavel

CHAPTER 9

Abandoned Twice

In third year Medicine I turned nineteen. Finally I was coping and felt relatively happy and settled. The year started out well for me. We had an influx of new students in our third year, who came from a Medical Science degree course. I fell in love, early on, with one of these students. His name was Hugh.

If I look back over my lifetime, I realise that this first love had the hallmarks of a 'true, first and only love'. Hugh was confident and enthusiastic, intelligent, dedicated and loved to study. He taught me how to study properly. I had struggled in the first two years and had failed a subject in each of first and second years, having to do supplementary exams during the Christmas holidays in order to pass onto the subsequent year. Hugh took me to the library with him each day after classes and taught me how to learn on a daily basis – and not wait till just before a test or an exam to study. We spent many hours studying together.

I had never before met anyone like Hugh. No one in my world had ever been respectful and responsive to my needs.

He was gentle and not pushy. I gradually began to trust him and to let down my defences. I opened my heart to him and began to come out of the frozen state I had been in. I knew with certainty that this was the man I wanted to marry. He was kind and patient and friendly and I was welcomed into his popular circle of friends, all from a northern suburbs background, so different from mine. He took me home to meet his parents in Sandton, a prestigious suburb where his father practised as a GP and his mother was a stay-at-home mum looking after her three talented sons. I felt out of place in this rich Jewish family but Hugh reassured me that his parents were liberal and open-minded and that they would love me as much as he did.

Hugh played the guitar in a three-man band which played in gigs all over Johannesburg on Saturday nights. He invited me along every time, and I sat spellbound, listening to songs of Simon and Garfunkel and other popular tunes of the day. I was 'Hugh's girl' and proud to be with him, the only one allowed to tag along with the band.

That year I learned to make my own dresses. Mother taught me to use her sewing machine and I was able to make lovely new dresses for the Saturday gigs. One in particular, a white dress, stands out in my memory as special. Hugh was always complimentary of my creative sewing skills.

Hugh and I were inseparable. My life was truly changing and I saw a future ahead, as his wife, in the northern suburbs, surrounded by friends and a big family. We talked about marriage after qualifying and were easy-going and confident, sharing our future dreams. I planned to get Mother fully better through my own expertise as a medical student, and looked forward to our classes in Haematology, where I would learn all about leukaemia.

The day finally came to begin Haematology. I can see the classroom clearly: long wooden desks with a microscope for each student, a set of slides alongside, and a textbook that accompanied the slides for each medical condition. Finally, there it was, the slide for leukaemia. I put it under the microscope and read the accompanying text:

Leukaemia is a group of cancers that usually begin in the bone marrow and result in high numbers of abnormal white blood cells.

Symptoms may include bleeding and bruising problems, feeling tired, fever, and an increased risk of infections. These symptoms occur due to a lack of normal blood cells. Diagnosis is typically made by blood tests and confirmed on bone marrow biopsy.

Treatment may involve some combination of chemotherapy, radiation therapy, targeted therapy, and bone marrow transplant, in addition to supportive care and palliative care as needed.

The average five-year survival rate is 57%.

My heart began to race as I grasped the information. Mother was now nine years post her announcement of having 'leukaemia, with twelve months to live'. I knew she hadn't had a bone marrow test nor any of the treatments mentioned. No chemotherapy or radiotherapy or anything that would at least give a prognosis of a 57 per cent five-year survival. She also did not have any of the symptoms listed in my book. I felt sick. I was confused and restless. I needed to get home to confront her and find out what was going on.

I did not, of course, share this with Hugh.

I arrived home that day shortly after 5 p.m. Mother was at the stove, cooking dinner. She had her back to me and greeted me casually without turning around. I noticed the whisky bottle and half empty glass beside her. I began by telling her that I had had an interesting day, that today we had started Haematology and that I had learned all about blood conditions. She didn't turn around and seemed uninterested. I said, 'Today I read about leukaemia, and what I learned is nothing like your illness. What exactly *is* wrong with you?'

My heart was pumping with anxiety. The air was thick with tension. My mother turned to face me and said, 'I have no idea what you're talking about!'

'But you told me you had leukaemia,' I said, 'and that you would die within twelve months. You told me when I was nine, after that braai here that Sunday...'

She got extremely angry and shouted, 'You are making this up! How dare you! I never said anything of the sort!'

At that moment, something cold and still filled my entire being. I turned around and walked quietly out of the kitchen. I went to my bedroom. I felt nothing. My body was cold and numb. My thoughts had ceased to be. I sat for hours on my bed, not moving. I remember waking up the following morning with my clothes still on.

I got up and carried on as if nothing had happened. My mother's denial was too big for me to handle. I put it away far, far away in a little mental box somewhere, not to be seen by me again.

My third year with Hugh continued to give me hope. I distanced myself from my mother and her issues as much as I could, but I was still conditioned to be helpful and considerate and I didn't know the meaning of 'No' when she made demands. Luckily my medical curriculum was very full and I was able to escape into what felt, by contrast, like a normal and happy group of friends. To me, Hugh's family were the epitome of what I wanted for myself one day.

Towards the end of third year I decided to spend the December holidays working at a youth summer camp. Hugh got me the job, as he had done this before himself, and he assured me that it was lots of fun. He had to accompany his family on their annual holiday down to Cape Town, he said, so we could not spend that time together. I missed him terribly.

I looked forward to our fourth year. The structure of medical training was to be very different. Our class of a hundred and ten students was divided up into 'Firms', groups of ten students each, who would spend the next three clinical years rotating through different subjects and a variety of hospitals, some as much as an hour's drive from the city. We chose our Firm partners carefully as we all wanted to get the best out of this close and shared experience. Hugh invited me to be in his Firm and I knew I would have the full support of a wonderful group of friends.

The entire class had to meet for the first day at Medical School to receive instruction on how everything worked and what the program was. Hugh was back from his holiday and had called me to ask if we could meet before class began the next day. I was delighted and got there early and waited for him. I thought we would go for coffee before the day started, but as he arrived in the corridor outside the lecture hall, I immediately sensed something was wrong.

He was serious and grim and did not smile as he came up. He told me we needed to talk and took me aside to a quiet part of the corridor. He said very quickly and earnestly, 'My father has told me to break off my relationship with you. He says I have to be in a different Firm from you. Because you are not Jewish, he says he will cut me off from my inheritance if I don't break off with you.'

I looked at Hugh's face and the expression I saw there made me realise immediately that this was something I could not fight. I'm not sure if I said anything at all. I think I simply walked away in silence. The rest of that day is a blur. I remember being put in a Firm with a random group of people who didn't know each other and seemed to be the ones left out. I could not have felt more abandoned, more betrayed, more unwanted.

I have often looked back at that 'after Hugh' time. For six months I cried into my pillow every night. During the day I hid my grief from everyone at home and at university. No one ever knew what a loss this had been and how much I missed him. I think I became walled off after that. I wasn't interested in relationships with anyone, not to any depth.

I managed to create a wall so high around my heart that I wasn't able to feel love, or warmth or tenderness. I completed medical school and graduated in December 1970. On a personal level I remained detached, in my head, distant. Life had simply given me one too many knocks.

As far as my medical studies went, I applied myself conscientiously in the final three years. I found a new purpose – being able to help the sick and the suffering. I decided that I would dedicate myself to my patients.

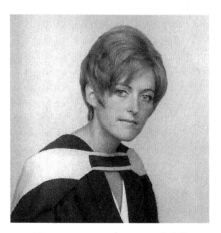

Me, at my graduation, 1970

CHAPTER 10

Doctor and Mother

From the time I qualified as a doctor in Johannesburg in 1970, I worked mostly at Baragwanath Hospital, situated in Soweto, south of Johannesburg. It occupies 170 acres, with 3,400 beds and over 6,000 staff members.

The Imperial Military Hospital, Baragwanath, was built in 1942 for convalescing British and Commonwealth soldiers. During the opening ceremony, Field Marshal Jan Smuts noted that, after the war, the facility would be used for the area's black population. In 1947 King George VI visited the hospital and presented medals to the troops there. From this start grew Baragwanath Hospital (as it became known after 1948), reputedly the largest hospital in the southern hemisphere. In 1997 another name change followed, with the sprawling facility now becoming known as Chris Hani Baragwanath Hospital in honour of the highly popular South African Communist Party leader who was assassinated in 1993.

Much of my time was spent working in the Casualty section where, on weekends especially, we received many seriously wounded people. It was common to see patients with axes in their heads, knives in their chests, and blood and vomit all over the floor. Casualty shifts were twelve hours long, often without a break. It was exhausting and incredibly stressful to work this way, but we remained as a team, together creating a spirit of camaraderie which helped ease the load. I remember my time in Casualty being a mix of intense seriousness and plenty of light-hearted laughter when the work was done.

At the age of twenty-eight, in January 1976, I married John Francis. He was a thoroughly good man, sporty, and kind and caring. I had a deep sense that this was the man who would be a father to my children one day. We lived on a farm on the outskirts of Krugersdorp. I continued to work at Baragwanath Hospital until a key event in South African politics decided John and me that we wanted to leave the country.

That event was the Soweto Uprising, a series of demonstrations and protests led by school children in the black township of Soweto. On the morning of 16 June 1976, about 20,000 black students walked from their schools to Orlando Stadium to protest against having to learn through the medium of Afrikaans. It was a peaceful demonstration, well organised and supported by teachers.

On the march the students were stopped by a police barricade. Choosing an alternative route and singing songs, they continued towards the stadium. They waved placards with slogans such as 'Down with Afrikaans', and 'If we must do Afrikaans, Vorster must do Zulu'.

The police set a dog on the protesters, who responded by killing it. The police then began to shoot directly at the children. Among them was thirteen-year-old Hector Pieterson. A photograph by reporter Sam Nzima of the dying Hector being carried away by another student made global news and became the symbol of the Soweto uprising.

The police attacks on the demonstrators continued, and twenty-three people died in Soweto on the first day. Among them was Dr Melville Edelstein, who had devoted his life to social welfare in Soweto. He was brutally stoned to death by the mob. Reporter Peter Magubane later found his body with a note saying 'Beware Afrikaans is the most dangerous drug for our future'.

Emergency clinics were swamped with injured and bloody children. The police requested that the hospital provide a list of all victims with bullet wounds to prosecute them for rioting. The hospital administrator passed this request to the doctors, but the doctors refused to create the list, and recorded the bullet wounds as abscesses.

The total number of people who died in the uprising is often given as one hundred and seventy-six, with other estimates of up to seven hundred.

I was working at the hospital in Soweto at the time. I was shocked and appalled at dealing with dozens of injured and dying children. I also felt frightened, being in what felt like a war zone. The numbers of casualties arriving was overwhelming and we needed to call colleagues in to help. Bodies were everywhere, on stretchers, on the floor, outside waiting in the backs of ambulances. Many children died because we were unable to get them to theatre in time to remove bullets or stop the bleeding. We worked through the night and I finally set off for home at 3 a.m.

As I drove along the main highway from the hospital towards Johannesburg, my car was stoned by an angry mob lining the road. The first stone hit my windscreen, shattering it. In that moment something inside me shattered too. I was afraid. I realised that it mattered little what 'acts of mercy' I had engaged in for the past twelve hours; I too could be killed.

That day I said to John, 'We have to leave this country. I don't agree with the political system and I am afraid for my safety.'

When I became pregnant later that year, an estimated seven hundred school children had been killed.

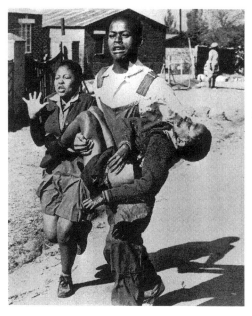

16 June 1976: the day Hector Pieterson died

We emigrated to the UK in early 1977. It was quite a culture shock and I was terribly homesick for South Africa. Living under grey skies with the constant drizzle of rural Cheshire was so different from my sunny Transvaal thorn bush and scrub.

Our first home was a flat in an old Victorian mansion in grounds abundant with flowering rhododendrons. A path led from the garden into the adjacent Delamere Forest. We acquired a border collie whom we named Penny Lane. Thus began for me long summer days of walking for hours in forests and fields with my sheepdog. I was ready to devote all my time and energy to my new life. Our son Simon was born in Chester in September and I became a delighted and committed stay-at-home mum.

A year later we bought our first small home, overlooking strawberry fields. I loved my role of mother and wife. I adored being able to read to Simon and to take long country walks with him. I enjoyed cooking and sewing and became quite good at restoring antique furniture. I attended auction sales and found old Welsh pine items of furniture which I stripped down in the garage. Despite missing the South African way of life, I was adapting to my new English home and enjoying the peace and tranquillity it offered. For me, being close to nature was healing and, even though this was not my beloved South African bush, it was green and lush – and safe.

I soon fell pregnant again, and in March 1979 our daughter Toni was born. I was overjoyed at having a daughter. I have vivid memories of the first few days in hospital, holding her and feeling that my heart was going to burst with love. When my obstetrician came in to check on my Caesarean stitches I told him that I was so happy, I wanted to have a large family! Having children was a heart-opening experience for me, beyond anything I had ever known or imagined possible.

Toni died. She was only four weeks old.

She had begun to vomit on day four, when still in the hospital. I was immediately alarmed. She was removed to the Special Care Baby Unit and investigated. She stopped vomiting and was discharged two weeks later, at the start of the Easter weekend.

With any medical problem, the system in the UK at that time was to consult your GP first. Toni began vomiting at home after her first bottle of the day. I was alarmed and called the GP when the second feed was also lost by projectile vomiting. The doctor assured me that to bring up milk, was 'normal' in young babies and that the problem was with me. He assured me that I was probably 'an overanxious mum'.

I refused to accept this and so he suggested that his nurse remain with me overnight and observe the feeding process and give me moral support. The vomiting continued and by morning my tiny baby was so dehydrated she was moribund. The nurse was deeply worried.

The GP was so shocked on his return the next day that he immediately ordered an ambulance to take the baby to Liverpool hospital special care unit, some thirty miles away. John, Simon and I followed the blue-light ambulance in our car. It was a nightmare scenario. From Toni's first vomit, I had had a gripping tightness in my solar plexus that did not let up. Not for one minute. I knew there was something terribly wrong. Yet I could not make the doctors believe me until it was too late.

The next twenty-four hours at the intensive care unit at Liverpool remain a blur. We sat in the bleak empty visitors' room while resuscitation was attempted. When we were eventually allowed to see her, Toni was lying on a slab with drips and tubes and machines attached to every part of her tiny body. It was awful to see. I stood at the door of the ICU looking on in horror. I wanted to run across and grab my baby off the slab and hold her. I could only turn towards John and bury my head on his chest and sob. I knew she was dead.

The paediatricians were unable to revive Toni sufficiently for surgery. She had gangrene of the bowel which needed surgical resection. She died on Easter morning.

Today, the seventeenth of March is her birthday. She would have been thirty-eight years old.

I shut down emotionally when Toni died. I seemed to drift off, right out of my body and far away. I was numbed out with shock. When the undertaker came around to the house and I opened the door to him, I was bewildered when he said, 'We have done such a nice job on her; would you like to come and see her in our Chapel of Rest?'

I almost slammed the door in his face! I was outraged that he could ask this of me!

I don't remember much of the funeral, apart from the tiny coffin moving towards the incinerator.

After Toni died John and I grew quite distant from each other. I became chronically anxious and hyper-vigilant. I had nightmares and flashbacks of my baby being rushed to hospital. I was fearful that something would happen to my other child. I wanted to share my fears with John but he seemed more and more removed from me and unable to discuss my fears. His job was also very demanding and he was struggling with his own stress at work; I did not want to create an additional burden. I took to drinking alcohol each evening. Often I would need four or even six cans of beer to be able to fall asleep.

The solution to my marital unhappiness, said my doctor, was to have another child. And so, two years later, our son Seth was born in Liverpool by Caesarean section. Having chosen the name Seth intuitively, I was very moved when told later that the name means 'compensation for the loss of a child'.

The doctor's advice was incorrect. Having this child did not make my anxiety and loneliness disappear. Nor did it bring John and me any closer together. Despite being overjoyed with my beautiful baby, I was extremely fearful that he too would die. The stress at home was becoming unbearable. I felt very alone with both children, and the fear of something bad happening to them continued. I lacked the confidence to reach out to anyone for help or support. Health visitors came and went, yet I remained silent. I was ashamed of not being able to cope on my own.

I couldn't understand what was wrong with me. The situation continued for a further three years. I was desperately lonely, afraid and ashamed. I kept a mask on and no one, not even John, knew how miserable I felt inside.

Eventually I decided that the only solution was for me to go back to work. If I could distract myself totally from my anxiety, I thought, I would manage better at home. I found a wonderful, full time 'grandmother nanny' for my children and, when Simon was eight and Seth four, I entered a four-year full-time training for General Practice. It would mean attending a hospital rotation scheme in the Liverpool area, a good two hours from home by car.

Thankfully John was willing and able to be there for the boys at night and on weekends, the times when I was mostly on call at the hospital. For this I am ever grateful. I am deeply sad though that I missed out a lot on the younger years of my two sons and that my marriage never did regain its closeness.

I graduated as a GP in 1988 and was offered a prestigious position as a partner in a country medical practice.

Having been immersed for years in medical training helped me to achieve some semblance of self-respect and confidence. The relationship between John and me, while no longer intimate, was friendly enough. My sons were well looked after by their nanny, and by the time I reached forty I thought I had achieved all my goals and dreams. I thought I had arrived!

Yet I had a nagging sense that something was still very wrong: despite all these achievements, I carried a deep inner emptiness.

And something else happened that I found disturbing. Not long after settling into my job as a country GP, I reached a critical point of impatience. One morning I had had a run of difficult, demanding patients, mostly talking about complex problems, and I felt out of my depth and unable to talk with them. I found myself thinking, 'If another patient walks through that door and complains, I'm going to scream!'

I was very disturbed by this strong negative reaction, the first of its kind I'd ever had. It was in stark contrast to the 'good bedside manner' that I had spent years cultivating. I knew I needed to get help.

Not long after, I saw an advertisement for Gestalt psychotherapy training in Manchester 'for the Helping Professions'. I sent for information and a booklet arrived. In it, Gestalt Therapy was described as 'The Process of Becoming AWARE'.

I had absolutely no idea what 'awareness' meant! I felt embarrassed and disturbed. *Awareness?*

Yet I was intrigued and could not put the booklet down – even when I was invited out for our annual hike with friends in Northumberland. The family went off without me and I remained glued to the little book, trying to grasp what it meant to be 'aware'.

I signed up for the year's training and the Gestalt weekly therapy that went with it. From the age of forty, through weekly relational therapy, I began to become aware. I started by uncovering the truth of my own childhood. Painfully, but courageously, I regained fragmented forgotten memories of betrayal, abuse, abandonment and despair.

I read many books, the most influential of them by the renowned psychoanalyst Alice Miller. In the 1970s she wrote about parental abuse, naming it 'poisonous pedagogy'. (The original German name was *schwarze Pädagogik* – 'black pedagogy'.) I gained insight into how my mother had manipulated and controlled me through her own narcissistic wounding. I started to understand how and why I had grown up disempowered and totally lacking in any feeling of self-worth. I also saw how steeped I was in shame.

For the next ten years I engaged in intensive weekly therapy. In 1998 I began training to become a Gestalt psychotherapist at the Manchester Gestalt Centre. After completing a year's course designed for people qualified in the helping professions, I decided to enrol in a Gestalt psychotherapist diploma course in Chester, running from 1990 to 1994. In 1996 I assisted with the Gestalt Diploma Training Programme in Bristol under Marianne Fry, Jenny Mackewn and Malcolm Parlett.

What was crucially healing for me through the Gestalt therapy process was being heard; being seen; being accepted and held in my pain and shame – without judgement.

Through the healing relationships I had with key Gestalt therapists, I began to regain my trust in people. It was slow at first. It took two years before I could feel the beginning of a connection with my therapist, Peter, and be able to receive his direct gaze. I had previously been unable to sustain eye contact with anyone in front of me, as I feared rejection. Regaining connection was a very slow process for me. After eighteen months of weekly therapy, I managed to look Peter directly in the eyes for the first time – and saw only compassion and kindness. It felt as if a knife was piercing my heart, and something inside me opened up. A little.

Soon I grew to trust others as well, mainly friends on the Gestalt training. With them I finally felt safe. My anxiety decreased considerably. I felt I belonged, at least to this community.

Being a Gestaltist became my way of life. I based my way of living on the Dialogic Gestalt Principle of 'respectful equality of acceptance, without judgement'. I applied this in my personal and professional relationships. At home and at work I became more functional. I was happy enough. The inner 'empty hole' was less noticeable. It was still there, but I managed to keep it at bay by working hard and remaining active. I was a successful GP and a successful Gestalt therapist. My life was as full as I believed it possible to be. Both my sons were growing into promising young men, and Simon was due to leave for university in the autumn.

And then suddenly, after my fiftieth birthday in 1998, John left me. Our marriage had been breaking down and this had been a long time coming. But I had been unwilling or unable to see it. When it happened, it felt sudden and brutal and shocking. The divorce came through later that year.

The grieving process that followed for the next two years tapped into what felt like a well of grief that held all the losses in my life, from childhood onwards. I did not fully understand it at the time, but with hindsight I know that this was a necessary part of healing. Thanks to my ten years of Gestalt, I was able to cope with it.

CHAPTER 11

Post Divorce: Return to South Africa

In June 1998, Simon, Seth and I, and our dog Ellie, left for Johannesburg. Seth had completed O levels and Simon was at Newcastle University and able to be with us during holiday times. My family in Johannesburg helped me to find a home and settle in. They all had problems of their own and I felt I could not impose on them too much. I was able to see my dear friend Sue of course, and we spent many long hours sharing what had become of our lives. Sue had lost her husband to cancer at the age of thirty-five and had been a single parent ever since. It was good to have one close friend to share with again.

As a support for my grieving process, I decided that what I most needed was a trip to Umtentweni on the South Coast of Natal. I bought a car and a trailer and before Simon returned to university we set off to the south coast – a good eight hours' drive from Johannesburg. I was excited to share the family 'shack', as we called it, with my sons. It was pretty run down, yet it still seemed magical to me. The avocado tree standing outside the hut had grown enormous and vervet monkeys were swinging in its branches, much to Ellie's delight.

The beach at Umtentweni was exactly as I remembered it: the small kiosk selling ices and sweets and tea; the stretch of beach sweeping across to the ocean with waves crashing noisily on shore. The smell of salt and sea evoked such a feeling of joy in my soul that I said to myself, 'This, *this* is home.' Each day I walked for hours and hours, feeling the waves wash away the sadness of my losses. The evenings together around the camp fire, with Cuban music filtering through the trees at sunset, were everything I needed to find myself again.

Each day I made footprints along the water's edge and I felt at one with nature. I kept upbeat during the days but returned to grieving after dark, once the boys were asleep. For months I had been grieving, a loud belly-howl coming from deep within. I had been told that this was necessary if I was to come 'through the other side of grief' and be truly healed and have my heart opened up. But I wasn't willing to cry in front of Seth and Simon, so I kept my grief confined to the early hours.

My grieving went on for two years. Then one day, at breakfast, Seth asked me, 'When are you going to stop crying in the night?' I felt terrible; I hadn't known he could hear me. I stopped crying then – at least so loudly.

We managed to have other special holidays during the two years I was back in South Africa. Each time Simon came home I took the boys, and often their friends as well, to places that were special to me from childhood. We hiked in the Drakensberg mountains and we camped in the game parks.

All of these touched a deep and essential place in my soul. I knew I was beginning to heal.

One of these holidays was especially transformative for me. I saw an advertisement in a newspaper entitled 'Tell Me Something I Can't Forget'. It was a writing retreat in the Kalahari Desert which included ten days of creative writing and meetings with the local Bushmen (now often more properly known as Khoikhoi or Khoekhoen[6]), whose custom it is to tell stories. I was hooked. In April 1999, I flew on my own to Cape Town and joined the group for the two-day road trip to the desert in an old bus. I was expecting an opportunity for creative writing. In actuality, I was to face a life-long mistrust and fear of women.

As we set off in the bus from Cape Town, I sat alone in the back seat and counted twelve women. Twelve! And no men. OMG.

I felt extremely anxious at first and grateful that I was left alone. It was a slow journey and eventually I began to relax. After a day the organiser came to sit next to me and shared why she had created this workshop. A close lawyer friend of hers had been fighting a legal battle on behalf of this particular Bushman tribe, whose land had been taken away from them by the South African Government. They had been removed from their nomadic desert life and land, and put into a small

---

[6] These terms have been under discussion in frequent years and little unanimity appears to have been reached. The words 'Bushman' and 'Bushmen' are therefore used throughout this book for the sake of simplicity.

fenced-in area of less than an acre. They lived in tin shacks like all squatters do. The three facilitators were co-writing a book about the plight of this tribe, and had already visited them several times. They wanted the world to know what had happened to this ancient culture now on the verge of extinction.

We travelled gently through different landscapes, moving from green mountains and forests to smaller bushy plains, until eventually we entered the Kalahari desert. I was struck by the amazing colour of the sand under the setting sun – a thousand shades of red. My companion turned to me and said, 'The desert with its exquisite lines and folds reminds me of a sensual woman. It turns me on when I'm here; I connect to the primitive in myself.'

I moved away from her after that, not sure if I wanted to hear any more.

As we eased our stiff bodies off the bus on arrival in darkness at 10 p.m., we claimed our rooms and paired up without any planning. I was thrown by the lack of structure: no rules and no explanations, and wondered how on earth I would cope in such a disorganised situation.

This Kalahari experience was the beginning for me of understanding what it means to allow a process to unfold organically and naturally!

At 5 a.m. the next day, before dawn, we were woken by Sakkas, one of the course facilitators (they gave themselves Bushman names). She invited us to join a ceremony to 'welcome the sun'... What? 'Oh well,' I thought, 'I'm awake now, I may as well join them.' In the dim light of approaching dawn I could make out the house where we were staying, a rambling single-storey with a large porch wrapped all around it. There was nothing else, just desert stretching into the distance.

We followed Sakkas, who looked like an American Indian with robes, a dark red tan, and tattoos all over her body. She said, 'Step only in each others footsteps, to spare the earth.' We stood in a semicircle, facing the direction of the rising sun, hands at our sides, palms open, waiting. It was freezing cold. But as the sun rose above the clear edge of the dune, she said a prayer, inviting energy into us. I felt myself warm up and in a few minutes we were flooded with bright, gentle morning sunlight. It was wonderful.

My fear of the women began to fade as I realised that they connected as deeply as I did to nature.

In our first morning circle, warmed by the rising sun, we were invited to share something about ourselves. We chose Bushman names to have for our time there. I was named 'Lego' by the women when I shared that I wanted to learn how to *let go* of past hurts.

Ever since childhood I had struggled with embracing femininity. I needed to allow myself to belong to a group of women who looked and behaved like *real* women. And the next step would be to be accepted by them. I dressed differently from them, in jeans and T-shirts, in browns and greys, while they wore flowing sarongs and scarves and brightly coloured beads. I felt apart, yet had no inclination to join them in dress.

Being in the desert had a huge impact on me. I would wander off alone to do my writing. I sat looking out at the timeless dunes while soaking up the smell of the earth, the scrub, the intense heat of the sun. Time seemed slowed down until it stood still. For the first time in my life I became aware of time as *eternity*.

We moved slowly, following a gentle group energy which flowed into each next phase of work, perhaps trance dancing, or making albums out of magazine scraps... The rhythms of nature from sunrise to sunset led the shape of the day, as it does with the Bushmen. After a while this organic rhythm touched an inner cord in me that felt feminine.

We visited the group of Kalahari Bushmen in their fenced-in camp. There were about forty of them, rounded up like the wild animals in the neighbouring game reserve, for economic gain. We found the group of adults known to our writers sitting under a thorn tree at the river. They were in traditional dress, loin cloth only. They welcomed us enthusiastically, with delight and much hand-clapping. We sat down and made a larger circle in the shade of the tree and they continued talking to each other. For the Bushmen, the most important aspect of their lives is relationship. They spend every moment they have, day and night, in conversation. Everything gets processed until it feels resolved. It is a matriarchal society. The women take gentle leadership and the men follow, be it talking or dancing or singing. Everyone collectively looks after the children.

I was struck by their total lack of bitterness about their huge loss of freedom to wander nomadically and to live off the land. What they shared was a deep sadness and acceptance, 'This is life,' they told me, 'we get on with it.'

As the week unfolded I longed to get out of my tight dark clothes and so I asked if anyone could lend me a sarong. Within minutes I was laden with beautiful scarves, sarongs and beads, generously shared. One of them said, 'Keep it, it looks lovely on you!'

From then on I wore flowing greens and yellows and reds and blues and I felt feminine. Someone said I had transformed into a beautiful butterfly.

On the last day we went high up on the dunes behind our house, to take photographs. Someone suggested that we should roll down the dunes, and for that we needed to take off our sarongs and scarves. Suddenly, there we were, all twelve women, naked in the sun and playing, laughing and rolling down the dunes.

We had a final photograph of us creating a mandala.

This experience had a lasting impact on me. I returned to Johannesburg feeling confident and centred. And a little bit more feminine.

CHAPTER 12

A Shocking Discovery

As I write my story, I see that my own healing was inextricably linked with attempts to heal my patients. Before I left England, I was already looking for 'another way', a better way, to work with patients, one that would bring about full healing. My own story would not be complete without sharing the story of Kate (name and details are altered).

I had known Kate, as her GP, since she was sixteen. When I first met her, she was recovering from a suicide attempt, an overdose, and I needed to visit her at home. Her parents lived in a council house, both were out at work and I saw her on her own. What struck me was how sullen and angry and silent she was. I felt out of my depth. I did not have the communication skill or ability to get through to her. Kate visited me regularly at the surgery, always unhappy, angry and unwilling to talk much. The inadequacy I felt during these consultations was a factor that drove me to take up Gestalt training.

Three years later, at the age of nineteen, Kate was diagnosed with nocturnal epilepsy. This meant that she had seizures, but only at night, while she was asleep. Hospital tests remained inconclusive and EEGs were negative for epilepsy. She was nevertheless put on anti-epileptic medication and stripped of her licence to drive. She consequently lost her job and was now at home, looking after the house for her parents. She was even more angry and railed at the unfairness of life.

By this time I was underway in my Gestalt training and had made it known at the practice that I would occasionally see clients for short-term counselling. One morning Kate came to see me to ask if she could have counselling. She said she was to be a bridesmaid at a cousin's wedding some months later and that she was too fearful to go out into a crowded public venue. She said she felt ugly and was too nervous to perform the part. Yet she desperately wanted to. After supervision advice, I decided to see Kate at my home for weekly Gestalt therapy. With counselling, she recovered enough to attend the wedding and afterwards asked if she might continue therapy with me. Her commitment, including the effort to get a lift to see me each week, made me agree. I have always been willing to 'go the extra mile', especially when met with such personal commitment.

Slowly Kate began to trust me. I still had no idea why she had attempted suicide at sixteen, but she was becoming less angry and more accepting of her life as it was. What I noticed however was that although our sessions took her 'one step forwards' in her feelings of self-worth, she would move 'one step backwards' during the interim time at home, where the environment was punitive and unsupportive. We continued with weekly therapy and what felt like a 'holding pattern', making little progress over the next seven years.

Then I was to leave the country. I began saying my goodbyes to my therapy clients several months before leaving. I sat with Kate in one of our sessions as she related the familiar sliding backwards that had occurred the preceding week. Suddenly I thought, 'Take her with you! She can live with you and have counselling all the time.'

Much to my surprise, Kate accepted the suggestion.

She had never been out of the country, nor on an aeroplane. My GP partners and her parents were supportive of the idea and helped raise the capital to get her to South Africa. She arrived shortly after us in Johannesburg and soon became part of our family. My sons were incredibly warm and accepting. Although Kate was twenty-six, she seemed to us like a young sixteen. The boys took her under their wing and she began to trust them. I didn't schedule any formal counselling sessions but chose to 're-parent' her, a therapy I had read about in the United States. She became my 'daughter' and I gave her as much love, respect, time and attention as I gave my own sons. We did things together and she shared our holidays. We took her to Umtentweni – it was the first time she had seen the ocean. She sat down and cried.

One night, not long after our arrival in Johannesburg, I heard screams coming from her room. It was past midnight. I rushed in expecting to have to deal with an epileptic seizure.

What I saw as I switched on the light was something else. She was asleep and squirming in the bed, screaming, 'Get off, go away, go away! No, no, no, no!'

I tried to wake her up but she was delirious. She was clearly having a terrifying nightmare. I sat comforting her, rocking her gently and saying, 'It's all right; you're safe now.'

We talked afterwards until she was settled enough to go back to sleep. She was reluctant or unable to mention the nightmare.

It happened again, regularly: screams in the night from her room, my finding her screaming 'No, no, no, no!' … and then her waking up in a sweat, terrified, shaken, and bewildered.

After several weeks of my being witness to this, Kate started to talk to me. Little by little the story came out. She had been terrorised as a young girl of sixteen when she was working as a farmhand, far away from home. She was locked up, beaten and raped. Repeatedly. Eventually she attempted suicide with a paracetamol overdose which resulted in her being admitted to Casualty for a stomach pump. Her parents were informed and her mother decided to take her home. That was how she managed to escape. She had been too terrified to speak about it, believing that her life would have been in danger if she told anyone.

I realised that Kate was not epileptic but suffering from PTSD, Post Traumatic Stress Disorder. Nightmares of this nature are a consequence of post-traumatic stress and can go on for years. They are often misdiagnosed as nocturnal epilepsy.

From then onwards I began to work with her through the lens of understanding her trauma. I worked with what had happened to her, in all its shocking detail. She needed to build up trust in herself and the world, and to feel safe again.

Knowing she wasn't epileptic, I allowed Kate to drive my car, a great boost to her confidence and self-esteem. Eventually she came off all medication, and her nightmares and anxiety faded.

Kate healed so thoroughly and so quickly, that within eight months she was ready to return to the UK, to a new and full life. Compared to the seven years of weekly counselling, this was a rapid and miraculous recovery. I was delighted for her.

I learned from this experience that I needed to follow my instincts when I had an idea for 'another way'.

Soon after our arrival back in Johannesburg I had found employment as a locum casualty doctor in a private city hospital. It was near my home – a small house I bought for my family, which included a dog and cat. We were happy there.

I enjoyed being back in a hospital role but soon realised that my surgical and emergency skills were rusty. I had spent far too many years focusing on Gestalt psychotherapy and had had little contact with trauma. The hospital sent me on a course in Traumatology and sixteen weeks later I was certified as a traumatologist, able to handle any emergency that came through the doors.

This was just as well, as the situation in Johannesburg was getting more dangerous. No longer did I experience the camaraderie and hope that people had held for the Rainbow Nation when Nelson Mandela began his presidency. Now, several years on, his promise of a shared future remained unfulfilled for the majority of South Africans. In its place a growing restlessness and frustration simmered in those who still lived in their thousands in tin shanties on the outskirts of the city.

Hijacking of vehicles was on the rise, as were armed robbery and violent crime. To protect themselves, many Johannesburg suburban communities created 'secure complexes' with high walls and armed guards. In Casualty we regularly dealt with gunshot wounds, burns and assault injuries. It was beginning to feel like Baragwanath in the seventies again.

I worked with a skilful team of trauma nurses who helped lighten the seriousness of what we dealt with each day. Our humour and ability to laugh at ourselves and with each other went a long way towards making a difficult job easier. I was a different person now, especially after my Kalahari experience: I was more sensitive and more connected to my feelings. The stories I heard and the emergencies I dealt with often reduced me to tears. I felt overwhelmed by the amount of suffering and by how little I was able to do to relieve it. I noticed that, like most of my colleagues who worked as 'first responders', I was living on a litre of Coca Cola and a pack of cigarettes a day. I also often consumed a carry-pack of six beers at night, to help me sleep after my twelve-hour shift.

Then one experience on a night shift became a turning point for me and I decided it was time to move on.

It was almost midnight on a Friday night. I was the sole doctor on in Casualty, with one senior nurse. We had finished the evening's work and were relaxing with a coffee when we heard an ambulance arrive. Rushing out with a stretcher to meet it, we were told that this was a burns case. A young woman had had petrol thrown over her by her husband and been set alight.

The hospital I worked in was a private hospital. Their policy in Casualty was to receive emergencies and, if patients were unable to pay, then we had to send them by ambulance to the nearest available government hospital for treatment. We were not expected to do more than the minimum resuscitation, as one might do at the roadside. I ordered that the patient be brought into the emergency room. She was conscious and, on my assessment, had 80 per cent burns, covering almost every part of her body. She told me her name was Precious. The nurse was already speaking on the phone with the burns unit at Baragwanath, some forty miles away. They were over-full on their burns ward and would not be able to take her. We would have to try other hospitals in the outlying areas, much further away. Looking at the woman who lay there quietly, I knew she would not make it if we had to do that. Without radical fluid replacement, she was likely to die. I instructed my nurse to get two units of plasma and to prepare for full fluid replacement right away. This was against hospital regulations. Together the nurse and I put intravenous lines up with plasma into both of Precious's arms. We began to dress her burns with layers of protective medicated dressings to minimise fluid loss and prevent infection.

I went ahead regardless of the expense incurred and the hospital regulations. At one point Precious turned to me, asking, 'Why are you helping me like this?'

I didn't know what to answer. She had overheard my arguments with administrators and my decision to break the rules. I was silent. It was impossible to voice the mixture of anguish and shame I held over the white privilege I enjoyed... so I simply smiled at her, wordlessly, and carried on doing my best for her.

She was taken by ambulance later that night to some far away hospital in the country, probably without skilled staff or adequate facilities. Precious went her to fate as a young black woman, facing death.

I walked outside, my heart heavy... and lit another cigarette.

In spite of regular holidays, I was getting run down by the stress of the work and the long twelve-hour shifts. In January 2000 I eventually became sick.

One morning I didn't show up for work at 7 a.m. The nurse on duty in Casualty called me at home. I was incoherent on the phone and she immediately sent an ambulance to fetch me. I was admitted with an extremely high fever. I was sweating and shivering as well, and it was thought I had malaria. I was put in an isolation ward. For three days I remained delirious and on the fourth day I regained some level of consciousness. All tests were negative for malaria and other tropical illnesses. It was a mystery.

As I lay in my hospital bed I came to realise I had had enough. The two years of struggling to make ends meet and of working with such awful suffering, had become too much for me. I decided that I did not want to go on living.

Suddenly I heard a commotion at my door. It was dark; way past midnight. The light went on and there was my son, Seth, coming towards me. I saw it was 3 a.m. and asked him what he was doing there at that time of night. 'I came to check on you,' he said, 'I felt worried about you!'

Seth sat next to my bed until daylight came through the blinds, when he said he needed to go home to shower but that he would be right back. It was my birthday and I was fifty-two years old. I had this amazing feeling all of a sudden that everything was going to be alright. I felt very much better – so much better that I sat up in bed and announced to the nurses that I wanted to go home.

Seth returned after breakfast with a birthday gift for me, a poem that he had written and framed himself. I was totally speechless. I realised, looking at my son, and taking in what he had written, that life was definitely worth living. I began packing my bag to go home. It felt as if my two years of grieving had finally ended.

CHAPTER 13

A New Marriage

After my high fever in early 2000, I returned to working in Casualty. But I was struggling with a financial crisis brought on by missing several weeks of work, and this made me decide to return to the UK to do some locum work. Simon was soon to return to South Africa permanently having completed his degree. Seth was doing catering work and both my sons told me that they wanted to stay in South Africa. I assured them I would only be gone for six months.

And then, serendipitously, I met Lawrence Dreyer during a workshop we attended on Valentine's Day, 2000, in Johannesburg. We became friends instantly and that same week Lawrence invited me to his flat for tea. He was a sixty-year-old 'confirmed bachelor' who had spent twenty-five years living in the East. He lived alone, Japanese style, in his flat in Killarney. I was a bit bemused on the first visit when asked to remove my shoes on entering the flat. I had to sit on the floor as he did not own furniture. He served tea in a black cast iron Japanese tea pot, accompanied by a beautiful little cake.

I realised that this man was as far removed from my medical mainstream life – existing on cigarettes and beer – as it was possible to be.

Then he asked me about myself and I began to share my story. I seemed to talk for hours, relating the journey I had travelled since Toni's death. He sat quietly and listened without interruption. Finally, he leaned forward and said, 'I see you, Melanie.'

I was taken aback. I'm not sure I'd ever heard this expression, apart from in therapy perhaps. He asked me if there was anything he could assist me with and I confessed that I didn't have enough money to get through to the end of the month. He laughed, saying he had never met a doctor with no money! He lent me R500. That was how our friendship began.

Within two weeks I'd invited him to come with me to the UK, as my friend and support. He accepted without hesitation, and set about selling his home and folding up his business. I organised for Simon and Seth to move into a secure complex, leaving all my household possessions with them. On 16 June 2000, I flew to England to begin my locum GP job in the Midlands, and Lawrence followed two weeks later.

Trauma occurs from a rupture in relationship, leaving in its wake a problem with trust. After my divorce I was extremely wary of ever having a relationship again. When I met Lawrence, I was willing to enter into friendship as this felt safe enough. I had been very lonely – lonely because I was not sharing myself at any meaningful level. Being with Lawrence was a unique experience for me. He provided a constant equal and respectful presence. He was always there for me.

Once we had settled in England, Lawrence decided that he would step into the role of 'house husband'. It made financial sense for me to work as a GP as I could earn much more than he would have been able to as a check-out assistant at Sainsbury's. (He did apply!) It wasn't easy for him, and we talked at length about the role reversal and the need for adjustment on both sides. My relationship with him provided an entry into a level of intimacy that hitherto I had not known.

A year later we decided to get married. We invited all the friends we had in England to our ceremony on the Easter weekend – which included a two-hour journey on the Severn Valley Railway steam train! We celebrated in one of the carriages with champagne and strawberries, and invited the conductor to join us.

Lawrence and I spent nine years in England. During that time I worked in many different GP practices, doing locum work. We moved several times, from Bridgnorth in Shropshire to the southern counties, and finally to Essex, where we ended up in Frinton-on-Sea in 2009.

I had left England before I was able to complete my final Gestalt Diploma in Manchester. I enjoyed being back in general practice, although I did miss my Gestalt psychotherapy. In 2002, we were on a holiday in France, staying at an old castle outside a small village. I woke up early one morning, and lay in bed looking at the sunlight filtering through onto the stone wall of our room and was reminded of the incredible time I had spent on a two-week Gestalt residential therapy workshop in France in 1996. It had been at the summer holiday home of Marianne Fry, our trainer, in Chamonix. I had fallen in love with the entire setting, surrounded by sunflower fields. The idea of working from home as a Gestalt therapist, was born at that time and I knew that one day I would like to have a home and workspace like that. I told Lawrence the story and he said, 'You have to go back to Gestalt. It's obvious you love it!'

On returning to the UK from our holiday, I contacted the Gestalt Institute of Cleveland, a major Gestalt centre in Ohio, USA. This was where Fritz Perls, the founder of Gestalt therapy, had worked. The Institute runs a two-year Gestalt Training Program for the helping professions. Lawrence and I both applied, and together entered an exciting and growthful journey, spread over twenty months and involving ten trips to the USA.

I made the most of being at Cleveland where so many excellent and well-known therapists worked. We attended workshops with people like Robert Lee, who was an expert and author on Shame. I believe my new ability to endure shame, and to recover quickly from a shame attack, was thanks to the powerful and enlightening weekend I spent with Lee. I was delighted with the more flexible and creative approach to Gestalt therapy of the Americans who taught us. This included learning to relate with horses! I noticed myself loosening up and becoming more open, more creative, more adventurous, and taking risks.

On each visit to America I had additional therapy with Jim Kepner, who wrote the book *Healing Tasks: psychotherapy with adult survivors of childhood abuse.*

Jim made a big impression on me. He was able to tune in to the gravity of the moment while remaining light in his approach. He readily self-disclosed and showed an unexpected humility during our time together. I was touched by his gentleness and kindness. I felt totally and compassionately accepted, as I am, all of me. I found myself trusting him very quickly.

One session with Jim was profoundly revealing and healing. In my diary in June 2004 I wrote:

I realise that my boundaries had been destroyed very early on. Which was why I had succumbed to sexual abuse at six. Jim suggested an 'experiment' for me. He offered me a blanket and asked me to wrap myself up in it where I sat on my chair. I did so and it felt good. I pulled it high up to my chin and was covered completely. He then started touching the edge of the blanket in a playful way, beyond my feet. I enjoyed laughing and pushing him away. Until he got closer. I began then to push his foot away and feel angry. He persisted playfully touching my feet through the blanket, encouraging me to respond. I got so angry I threw a cushion across the room. Suddenly a wave of fear washed over me. It lasted five minutes. I cowered, expecting a beating. He helped me to come out of the fear and to calm down, claiming my 'personal space' in the blanket. He said that I had done well, that I had claimed my space and that I WILL defend it in future.

This Body Process work, for which Jim is well known, was very powerful and transformative for me. I returned to England after that visit which included the session with Jim Kepner feeling that I could say 'No' and not fear punishment. It was to be a highly significant personal shift that would lead to a remarkable set of events over the next few months.

A few months previously, I had been offered a permanent GP partnership in a seven-partner practice in Sussex. Having searched widely for a practice I could align myself with, I was sure that I had found what I was looking for. They were rated as one of the top five medical practices in terms of their earnings and their performance. I was proud to be a second female partner in such a high-flyer environment. I was given my own list of two thousand patients, inherited from the retiring GP whose place I was taking. I had my own room, my own desk, and a new computer. I was all set to finally be a proper doctor, and my promising future was mapped out. Lawrence and I bought a house and began to take root in our new community. My diary at that time says:

I finally feel a part of the ground of England by choice. I feel supported, seen and valued.

I am happy, inspired, creative and free to be the kind of doctor I would like to be. I love the practice and the doctors and staff and patients. It's strange to see my name printed on stationery and scripts and the large letters above my door. When patients ask me,

'Are you my doctor?' it's thrilling to say, 'Yes!' I have thrown myself into the work and been incredibly thorough, giving each patient I see a full review and getting computer records up to date; I aim to do my best for every patient... I am taking root here in this town. I feel strong and stable and able to flourish and finally to bloom in my fullness. I can support others now without losing my groundedness.

I felt I was different at this practice. I was excited about consulting, excited to be the best I could be. I was aware that my ability to relate and communicate was excellent, and it was obvious that patients were receiving me well. I usually left the rooms long after the other doctors had gone home. On one occasion a senior partner came in to ask why I was still there at eight o'clock when the surgery had been closed since six. I shared my enthusiasm for reviewing each patient and the time I needed to make this investment. He warned me that I was 'overdoing things'. I was naturally shy and reserved so I continued quietly to do my own thing behind closed doors. A month or so after this, one of the receptionists confided in me that several patients had transferred onto my list from one of the senior partners.

About this time, one of my young male patients was diagnosed with terminal cancer. I visited him in hospital and continued terminal care visits at home, supporting his wife and young family. He died within a month. I did my best to support the grieving widow. I didn't know her as well as my patient, but understood her circumstances and was willing to do the frequent home visits she requested. Then she began to behave rather oddly. She got hold of my email address and started writing to me on my personal email. She wanted more from me than I had been giving, she explained; she wanted to meet for coffee and to go for walks. I felt out of my depth as a new GP trying to do my best for all my new patients. But this didn't feel comfortable. I agreed initially to a few such meetings but soon began to see that the grieving widow was emotionally unbalanced. I understood her problem, but I had to respect the boundary of the doctor-patient relationship.

Things escalated and she wrote desperate letters of need almost daily, begging me to meet with her. I said No and gave clear reasons why it was incorrect and unacceptable for me to do this as her doctor. I chose to hold the boundary, without responding to her calls or emails or letters dropped off at my house.

When I next was away in Cleveland for a week's training, she went to the senior partner and made a complaint. She told him I had sexually abused her. He was allegedly 'so shocked' at the allegation that he consulted with his partners immediately. They agreed to make an immediate complaint in writing to the General Medical Council (GMC). They chose not to wait for me to come back and answer the complaint.

On my return to work the following Monday, I was met at the door of the surgery by the practice manager who asked me to hand her my surgery keys. She led me into a room where two of the partners were waiting. They interrogated me for an hour and I told them exactly what had happened and how I had managed the situation. I said I believed the woman was emotionally unbalanced and I totally denied the allegations.

However, they said it was too late to do anything as they had already sent in the complaint and it had been accepted by the GMC. They said they had been ordered to suspend me as I was 'guilty until proved innocent', according to medical law. I was suspended from working as a GP – on full pay for the next six months, while being investigated. After that I would be without a job. I was told not to speak to any member of staff nor any patients at any time under any circumstances. I was dismissed.

I went home that morning to Lawrence. I barely explained what had happened before I crawled into a foetal position in the corner of my couch and remained silent. I retreated inwards so far that for several days Lawrence could not get me to talk or to eat. I simply sat there. What I was running through in my 'frozen state' was an imaginary court case. I pictured myself being found guilty and imprisoned. A male doctor I knew up north had recently been imprisoned for allegedly 'touching up' a woman while examining her for a whiplash injury. She won in court as there had been 'no third party witness'. It was her word against the doctor's and the courts nowadays favour the patient.

I knew I faced going to prison. I knew I had lost my job. I knew that my partners had betrayed me and I knew the widow had lied, in her unbalanced state of mind. Lawrence was enraged, and remained so for the next few years. He kept saying things like, 'I'd like to throw a grenade into the surgery and blow everyone up.' I was less angry.

In the twenty-seven months of my suspension, I began to create jewellery. I learned to make glass beads and use them to make beautiful necklaces and earrings. I eventually sold my creations to a shop in the town and managed to get quite a nice income. To this day, threading beads is my meditation time, the time in which my brain turns off, and I enjoy the colourful piece I am creating in the present moment. I have just today completed a necklace in shades of blue, turquoise and pink which I shall wear next week. The skill of being able to create beautiful jewellery is still a constant delight to me.

I had to earn money after my six months of pay came to an end. The GMC allowed me to work on the night call services. In the UK, GP patients are seen by an on-call service which operates seven nights a week, from 6 p.m. till 8 a.m. the next morning. The doctors are paid by the on-call service and taken to each visit by a driver. I was given permission to work in the Thames-doc service, provided I was accompanied at all times by a chaperone. This meant I wasn't allowed to see patients on my own as I was considered 'a danger to the public'. The chaperone was usually the receptionist on duty or the driver, both of whom had no experience of being witness to intimate medical examinations, sometimes with the patients undressed. It was embarrassing for them and humiliating for me. But at least I was able to survive financially.

Eventually my hearing took place on 24 November 2006 in London. It was a cold and grey day as Lawrence and I made our way to the court. Reporters were at the door and several took photos of me. It was awful. The courtroom was filled with reporters during the first half in which the defendant's barristers presented their case. I noticed that the reporters left after the first half and before my case was presented. They chose to have only half the story.

This is what I wrote in my journal:

> The hearing was everything I hoped for. The panel appeared wise and compassionate. One of them asked, 'How did this case get this far?' They commended me on my actions and said that in their opinion, the complaint had been a backlash, a result of me holding a boundary. I was exonerated. I was set free.

Lawrence was relieved, tearful and full of joy. We went home, exhausted after a long day. Early the next morning I had a phone call from a friend to warn me that I had made front page news in the local paper. There was a picture of me outside the court with the headline: 'The doctor, the widow and the lesbian kiss'.

I could have been mortified, taken down and deeply hurt. This did not happen. Going through this two-year suspension and complaint and facing the possibility of imprisonment, had radically changed me. I felt immensely strong, certain of who I was. And of who I am – someone I can face each day in the mirror, smiling.

We bought the paper that day and decided to put it on the pile for the fire.

We completed our certification Gestalt Training in Cleveland, fully and generously supported by the large group of American friends on the course. It was good not to feel alone with the drama, and we began to prepare for a four-week December holiday back in South Africa at the end of 2006. We planned a round-the-country trip with Simon and Seth. I was hoping to wash away what remained of the hurt and humiliation of the complaint.

CHAPTER 14

A New Direction

During our holiday in South Africa in December 2006 I realised how passionately I wanted to go home again. Walking on the Natal beaches and feeling the ocean speak to me, I knew that I was not finished with this country of my birth, this country of my suffering. I knew I would be living for the next few years in the UK with an ache in my heart for South Africa.

Back in the UK I explored a number of GP practices, and decided that Clacton-on-Sea in Essex was a suitable place for me to work. Upon applying, I was offered a part-time partnership in a practice in this small coastal town, and shortly after, a second one in nearby Frinton-on-Sea. Lawrence and I found a lovely home to rent in Frinton-on-Sea, just a few minutes' walk to the quintessential English promenade and seafront.

Initially I was fearful of returning to general practice. But I discovered I had changed during the intervening two years. To my surprise, I absolutely loved it. I noticed how much more sensitive I had become to my patients' suffering, and I could feel that I cared more than ever.

My patients in Essex were some of the most unhealthy I had encountered in decades of general practice. They were also the most stressed. The majority of families existed on social security support; many were jobless, and many mentally ill or alcoholic. A temporary caravan park had been set up on the seafront on the outskirts of Clacton and I visited my bed-bound patients there.

I was shocked to discover the levels of poverty and the awful conditions that people were having to cope with.

There were no roads in this area. The families were living on beach and marshland and I was always nervous when making visits because my car would often get stuck in the soft, wet sea sand. Social Services in many northern British counties had been sending their 'most difficult to manage' families down to Clacton, where they were effectively dumped in temporary caravans, until such time as more suitable, permanent accommodation could be found. This would take months, often years.

Stress was ubiquitous. Many of the men were veterans returning from the wars in Iraq and Afghanistan, suffering from Post-Traumatic Stress Disorder. Many were addicted to alcohol and drugs. Matt was typical of the patients I visited. I saw Matt on most Mondays following his discharge from hospital on the weekend, having tried yet again to kill himself. I felt absolutely ill-equipped to help him break the cycle of self-harm.

Another young patient, Pat, suffered from unstable diabetes that required insulin injections every two hours. Pat was deeply depressed, suffering from insomnia and chronic back pain. He was unemployed – and unemployable. Whatever help I was able to offer these forty-year-old men was ineffective in relieving their suffering – a story that was much the same for all my other patients.

The small town of Frinton, two miles away, was slightly more upmarket. It was primarily a retirement town for the elderly, and more than three quarters of my patients were over sixty years old. People retired to the quiet beauty of this seaside resort, drifting into old age homes and infirmaries in their later years. As their GP, I was faced with managing the multitude of chronic diseases they suffered from, and the associated polypharmacy. My home visits consisted of rationalising their medication, often sorting through twenty bottles or more of different prescription drugs to see which could be intelligently removed. Much of their ill health and current symptoms were due to drug side effects and drug interactions. To me it felt insane for them to continue on so many tablets.

Having previously worked as a GP only in middle class communities in other parts of England, I was not prepared for the levels of stress, illness and infirmity I was seeing in Clacton. What was clear to me was that patients in Essex were being diagnosed with life-threatening illnesses at younger ages than I had seen previously: heart attacks would occur when they were in their twenties; cancers such as breast cancer and bowel cancer, in their thirties. Many had chronic pain, arthritis and debilitating chest conditions. Most had mental problems, and almost all were taking anti-depressants, sleeping tablets or morphine-related painkillers. What was going on here? Why had I not seen this before in Cheshire or in Sussex?

I was curious, and began to ask my patients for their stories. I invested more time, with longer home visits, to sit and really listen to them. Between the end of morning surgery at 12.30 and the start of evening surgery at 4 p.m., I would make a point of visiting my patients at their homes. They enjoyed my coming round to their 'humble abode' and they would have a welcome cup of tea waiting for me and smilingly encourage me to sit in 'the most comfortable chair'. I even enjoyed taking the risky road to the caravan park, leaving my car at the nearby pub and walking barefoot through sea sand to the patients in their caravans and sheds.

I often felt overwhelmed by the magnitude of their suffering, as I listened in these quiet hours. What happened there was a very important realisation for me.

Every patient who shared their story described a difficult childhood, with many traumatic experiences, continuing as a theme throughout their early lives. As we sat with our tea, each one telling a similar, painful story, a picture started to emerge. I wondered if there was a correlation between the amount of stress they had experienced in childhood, and the appearance of early physical and mental illness.

Back at home, each evening Lawrence would listen to me sharing the issues of the day as I complained that medicine was not working. My repeated comment was, "There has to be another way!" And on one occasion he jokingly said to me, "That will be the title of your book."

What was becoming very clear was that I was stuck in a 'healing profession' that was not helping anyone to get better. The only good I seemed to be doing was when I took the time to create a genuine, caring relationship with my patients. And I knew I was walking a tight-rope with this tactic – it was a risky endeavour for me, having been punished through litigation back in East Grinstead only two years previously.

I wondered, almost daily: "*Is* there another way? What else could possibly work for these patients?"

In early 2008, a breakthrough came with a chance encounter.

Lawrence and I happened to be visiting a Constable art exhibition in a small nearby town when we spotted someone in the crowd who looked just like an old friend of ours from Canada. Of course it couldn't actually be our friend, so many miles from his home, in a small southern English town. Yet, unbelievably, it was! Ron visited us regularly in Frinton thereafter and I began to share some of my frustrations as a GP. I was beginning to wonder how much longer I could remain working as a doctor. Ron offered me a book that had recently inspired him, *The Biology of Belief* by Dr Bruce Lipton. It seemed a dubious title but, despite my scepticism, I read it.

Reading Bruce Lipton's work was a pivotal point in my life.

Lipton began his career as a cell biologist. As a professor of biology at Stanford School of Medicine, his research showed that the outer layer of the human cell was essentially an organic 'computer chip' which worked as the 'brain' of the cell. Furthermore, he showed that our environment, operating through the cell membrane, controlled the behaviour and the physiology of the cell. "It is the environment that turns genes on and off," he emphasised.

This astonishing fact led to the modern science of epigenetics. I learned, in short, that very few of our medical ailments are due to genetic inheritance – as had previously been thought. Only about six per cent of all medical conditions are genetically inherited. Everything else is created by our environment, acting on us at the cellular level to activate genes and influence our biology.

All of our thinking, whether positive or negative, has a significant impact on our biology. According to Lipton, if you believe you will get cancer and you hold a lot of fear around cancer, you will significantly increase your chances of developing it. For me, this was a revolutionary concept.

As a doctor I had been taught that medical conditions – even personality traits – were mostly inherited and passed down through genetics. I believed that we inherited bad genes and poor health.

Dr Lipton was describing the opposite: that we are able to influence our internal and external environments and therefore able to create our own state of well-being and health.

It is hard to describe what happened to me. A new reality, a different world opened up. I was thrilled, excited and exhilarated, knowing that our lives are under our own control and not subject to genetic inheritance.

This was the piece of the puzzle that finally allowed me to walk away from conventional medicine. I handed in my six-month notice at both surgeries, despite a fear of the economic hardship this would bring, and began researching the brain and the subconscious mind through neuroscience and neuroplasticity.

I attended every course and training in this field that I could get to. With a London-based specialist, I learned about working with the subconscious mind using a specific brain frequency called Gamma. In my final months at the surgery, I tested this method with a few of my patients. Almost to my disbelief, the results were astounding. I felt as if I had walked through a doorway into a different universe. Excited and hopeful, deep inside I knew this was the path I needed to take.

Everything I read, researched and trained in expressed a single thought – the need to work with the subconscious mind. It was powerful and alluring. Yet there existed, for me, a gap between the theory and the practice. Despite every method and modality I uncovered, I could not find a way to work with the subconscious that I believed was 'clinically usable'.

This combination of inspiration and frustration would act as the driving force behind the eventual development of my own method for working with the subconscious mind, a method I named 'Quantum Energy Coaching' (QEC).

PART 2

The Other Way

CHAPTER 15

Four years later

Here I am in Devon, England, looking out of my window onto a green lawn with daffodils, announcing an early spring. It is Easter weekend, April 2021. I have spent several days reading my story again. I've had to take it slowly, as reading about my life, especially as a child, is very moving. I am also aware of the many painful experiences I suffered as an adult, such as losing my daughter Toni on Easter Day, which makes tomorrow an important landmark. She would have been forty-two this year.

It is four years since I began writing my story, and twelve since I resigned from general practice.

These past twelve years, mostly spent in Cape Town, the last few in Spain and finally in England, have included an important internal factory experience of creative development and refinement of my own work, Quantum Energy Coaching.

As I take up the task of finishing this book, I am drawn to share my own healing with QEC. Many of you will be able to relate to parts of my story as my key traumas are common to many. There will be time ahead for me to write technical books on how QEC works, and offer books on patient case studies and how these have transformed lives. I could in fact write several books, as my life since leaving formal medicine has been richly centred around creating and developing this remarkable method. The stories are compelling.

Without using pharmaceuticals, without complex treatments or lengthy talk therapies, clients all over the world have transformed their lives through QEC. These are their words, not mine. Since lockdown, our QEC Practitioner Training has moved online and reached a wider population through the internet. I have worked with thousands of patients, and still do – with rapid and full recovery. QEC is reaching those who need it, thanks to our incredible, growing community of practitioners.

As I sit here today writing this chapter, I am finally ready to step up and shout out: " I have found another way!"

CHAPTER 16

The origins of QEC

Many of you reading this will already have experienced Quantum Energy Coaching yourselves. Perhaps some of you are certified QEC practitioners. However, before I share my own healing journey, I feel it important to explain, in essence, what QEC is, for those who are reading about it for the first time.

QEC was born from the crucible of Medicine and Gestalt Relational Therapy. Since my experience with the Kalahari Bushmen and their camp-fire story-telling, I've known that stories and relationships are key to healing. For me, any healing method – including medicine – which does not invest the time to tune in, listen, see and understand, is working at a far too superficial level.

With QEC we work to transform limiting self-beliefs, behaviour patterns and physical conditions – safely and quickly. A typical session begins with relationship and dialogue to define a client's unique needs by hearing their story. What follows is the QEC method, a combination of a variety of techniques that serve to work with the subconscious mind.

We create a Gamma frequency that allows the neuroplasticity of the brain to 'rewire' itself – dispensing with unhelpful belief systems from conditioning and past trauma. There is no meditation or hypnosis involved. The client is fully awake and aware, and in charge of their own healing process at all times.

Relationship and dialogue

Relationship in therapy is achieved through the Gestalt dialogic process and includes periods of intimacy in I-Thou moments, when therapist and client connect and meet one another, fully. This sacred experience is the essence of how Gestalt therapy heals: creating a trusting relationship to feel connected, then exploring issues and becoming aware of behaviours which the client may want to change. In Gestalt, awareness is considered a necessary step towards change.

This process facilitates an understanding of how the client has lived with his or her limiting thoughts or destructive behaviours. Once we have arrived together at an understanding of what the issues are, I empower the client to choose the change they want.

This is done through the metaphor of a miracle or magic wand – the ability for the client to choose their own solution in their own words.

For example, if a client tells me "I hate myself", I *could* respond with "What would you prefer to feel?" Most people would tell me "I wouldn't want to hate myself." The introduction of a 'magic wand' however, gives the client permission to access the highest form of imagination and creativity. Bypassing the restrictive influence of the 'practical' and the 'realistic' conscious mind, we're able choose a much more powerful statement, corresponding to our highest creative solution. With a 'magic wand' a client may instead say "I love and accept myself totally." This becomes the personalised sentence to 'install' into the subconscious mind using the Gamma Wave method later in the session.

Accessing the subconscious

In London in 2008 I attended several trainings with Dr Chris Walton, the developer of the Gamma Mindset. Gamma is the brain frequency that is most effective at creating transformative change in the subconscious mind. After learning the method, I began to test it on myself and, although I had some generally positive results, I was puzzled that the changes I experienced were not particularly accurate. After much analysis, I realised that the 'sentences' I was 'installing' were not unique to me and my history. I felt they needed to be. Coming from a Gestalt background, I was uncomfortable being asked to install into my own subconscious mind a list of new beliefs made up by someone else.

I was inspired to refine what was obviously a powerful tool by finding a way to work with the subconscious mind that would be specific to my unique story. I said goodbye to Chris and got his blessing to take the Gamma Mindset method and integrate it into whatever therapeutic process I could develop that would suit me better.

I now incorporate the principles of Chris Walton's Gamma Mindset in QEC as a simple and effective method to install new beliefs – unique to each individual – into the subconscious mind.

The many facets of healing

Traumatic experiences and the wounds they inflict are complex, nuanced and unique. To work with them requires a holistic approach that addresses each individual facet. The continued refinement of QEC in the field has developed a way of working that today is incredibly powerful.

During the past few years I have begun to work with what I call my 'QEC Trauma Formula'. Its key component is to offer forgiveness for what was done.

I was moved and inspired to work with forgiveness by Nelson Mandela. When he came into power, he set up the South African Truth and Reconciliation Commission with a number of other appropriate people, including Archbishop Desmond Tutu. The purpose of this commission was to provide the victims of apartheid a space to tell their stories – to be heard and be witnessed by the perpetrators of the atrocities – at a civil hearing. Victims were invited to share their stories and to receive a response from the alleged perpetrators, who in most cases, showed deep regret. The victims were invited to forgive, and there were no further legal actions. This extraordinary three-year process led to a peaceful transition in my country, previously gripped by decades of injustice and violence.

My experience has shown that this technique is able to achieve something that has not been easy with the other methods I have tried – the ability to wipe the slate clean of past trauma.

QEC will never stop evolving. Like 'open source' software, we will all contribute to the continued refinement of the method with an open mind, an open heart and an inquisitive soul.

CHAPTER 17

My own healing with QEC

I am writing this book for my community, for all of you have shared your stories with me over the past twelve years. In the preceding chapters I have shared my journey with you. What follows over the next four chapters is the story of my personal therapeutic work on my own core traumas. I have chosen four major life traumas that I worked with using QEC between 2017 and 2020 as these were the ones that had shaped me and created challenges for me throughout my life.

These four traumas occurred at different developmental periods of my life, and created a miserable existence for me as an adult. They were not alleviated with Gestalt talk therapy over two decades.

I'll share with you exactly how I used QEC to make a full recovery, so that I now enjoy a life of deep connection, joy and fulfilment.

CHAPTER 18

My first early childhood trauma

Growing up, I believed I had a normal childhood. In fact I actually felt that I was fortunate to have been born to such wonderful parents. I understood that children got smacked if they were naughty, and I thought myself lucky because the wooden clothes hanger didn't break when I got beaten by my father, as it did for my brother.

In truth, I had a distorted view of my childhood under the age of ten. When I entered therapy at the age of forty, I was totally convinced that my childhood had been better than most people's. The reality, as I have discovered, was very different.

My mother was twenty when she had me. Her own history, as I have mentioned, was one of abandonment, losing her own mother to alcoholism at age thirteen, and her father to work in distant Rhodesia. She only saw him for two weeks of the year. She was schooled in an abusive, punitive convent and lived with relatives who rejected her. Her uncle sexually abused her.

This did not lay a good foundation for managing the arrival of her firstborn child. She was totally frozen – a term used by neurologists to explain what happens in the autonomic nervous system (ANS) when exposed to severe or chronic trauma. Being frozen meant that she was emotionally disconnected and distant, living only in the intellect. This was my mother, and this was the person who tried to breastfeed me in the nursing home while being humiliated by a lesbian nurse. I was bottle-fed after that, and shame was ever-present when I was near my mother.

My early years consisted of complete emotional abandonment. Every photograph I have of myself is of me sitting alone – in a cot, a playpen, a chair or a pram. Not a single picture of being held, by anyone. With my father away at work for long hours, my mother was alone with me and apparently could not tolerate any form of emotional outburst. When I was a toddler I threw a temper tantrum on one occasion and she responded by trying to strangle me. I recalled this memory as an adult during Body Process Work with Jim Kepner in Cleveland. Being rejected, emotionally abandoned and almost killed put me into freeze by the age of three. I never again knew anger, and most of my other emotional states were muted. I understood later why I needed to split off from anger – it was life-threatening.

My mother hated physical contact and would push me briskly away if I got anywhere close to her. I soon got the message that I disgusted her, and I inevitably embraced the core belief that I was disgusting. I believed this was true about myself throughout my life, until I healed through QEC. It was a belief that remained unshakable throughout years of therapy, despite the obvious love and respect that I received from my therapists.

I never regained a connection with my mother.

This early trauma impacted me profoundly throughout my life. I was neurologically frozen, experiencing the world as if through glass. I felt lonely and disconnected from people, and even from life itself. Others experienced me as detached and aloof, and I was nicknamed 'The Iron Maiden' at medical school. I found it difficult to make friends and had a deep emptiness, an inner sense that something essential was missing. But I believed the fault was mine; I knew I was disgusting and unlovable.

I adapted by creating a false outer persona or mask – that of being available to help or be of service. I discovered early on that my parents gave me attention if I served them, and this quickly became my modus operandi. As 'mother's little helper' I found myself with a full-time job taking care of my three brothers and sisters. Being rewarded for doing so set the lifelong belief that the needs of others were more important than my own.

Starved of connection, I gladly gave up on all of my own needs – caring for the needs of others was the only strategy that got me the attention I craved. However, it left me unable to say No or to set boundaries.

By the time I became an adult, my anger was 'split off' – I couldn't feel it. I was therefore unable to gauge whether people were manipulating me, or if I had been wronged. I had a confused and emotionally flat response to what others saw as an outrage on my behalf. Often this would lead me to misjudge situations and I would find myself in many dangerous predicaments. It took eight years of Gestalt psychotherapy for me to slowly get in touch with my anger – and it was a frightening process.

From the age of nine I suffered from addictions. Dr Gabor Mate, renowned addiction expert, explains that the cause of addiction is early proximal abandonment (the experience of the primary caregiver being there physically, but not able to connect emotionally).

All traumas in a developing child (up to the age of seven especially) have a lasting impact on one's life. In fact they are considered by most of the medical and therapeutic professions as being very difficult to heal. I certainly knew that my eight years of Gestalt therapy, while helping me to get in touch with my anger again, could not change my deeply-held beliefs about being disgusting, unlovable and worthy only of service to the needs of others.

QEC work on my core, early childhood trauma

As an adult, I generally 'lived in my head', with little, if any, connection with my emotional world. After many years of Relational Gestalt therapy I was able to connect reasonably well with patients, friends and family that I trusted, but I noticed that I continued to withdraw after a short time of social contact. In fact, I used alcohol to withdraw from social contact, as being disconnected felt safer, more familiar.

It was clear that this addictive drive came on only when I was stressed or highly stimulated. Alcohol seemed to be almost like a calming medication that I had to have. The unwelcome consequence was that it shut me off emotionally at a time when I was beginning to really enjoy contact with those near and dear to me. Contact with my students, and my patients especially, had become rich and rewarding and I was beginning, over time, to be more able to sustain this without stress.

I wondered if my need to 'self-medicate' with alcohol would lessen of its own accord if I healed my other traumas. I made the decision to allow myself to continue using alcohol when emotionally overwhelmed, paying close attention to the nuances around this behaviour, so as to better understand it.

Everything I had previously been taught about addictions was wrong. As Gabor Mate explained in his book *In the Realm of Hungry Ghosts*, when our autonomic nervous system is triggered into its trauma pattern, we remain in an unpleasant, emotional over-charge for hours, or even days. A healthy, balanced nervous system recovers within a very short time, but a traumatised, dysregulated nervous system is easily overwhelmed and remains in stress.

For the first time, I truly understood that addiction is a human attempt to relieve or lessen the impact of intense, painful or overwhelming states of feeling. I was now convinced that to be free of my addictions, I had to fully heal all my past traumas. This would have the effect of balancing my autonomic nervous system, enabling it to return to healthy, natural homeostasis very quickly.

My first task with QEC, therefore, was to bring myself out of freeze, and out of the addictive cycle. I instructed my nervous system to return to optimal function. I also added a sentence to release background levels of anxiety and shame, in order to allow myself to remain in homeostasis.

These are the actual QEC sentences that I installed in 2017:

** My ANS is in optimal balance and homeostasis
** I release all levels of anxiety and shame
(*As you will see below, these two sentences were a necessary starting-point each time I used the QEC formula for a different trauma.*)
I forgive my mother her total inability to love and care for me and connect with me in the way I needed
I forgive my mother for passing her self-disgust and shame on to me
I forgive my mother for trying to kill me when I became angry, causing me to split off my natural anger-response for the rest of my life
I forgive my mother for narcissistically using me for her own needs at each and every turn, without any understanding or concern for the impact on me
I forgive my father for his absence and his ignorance in leaving me in the dangerous and damaging care of my traumatised young mother
I forgive myself for any part I played in this trauma
I release all terror, fear, anxiety, despair, confusion, hopelessness, emptiness, loneliness, grief and anger as well as all toxic shame, related to this trauma

119

I restore trust in myself to 100% on all levels

I restore my internal safety to 100% on all levels

I am a beautiful, lovable woman, worthy of love and worthy of existence, on all levels

I am free of disgust and replace it with sacred, inner self-respect

I embrace my capacity for anger and enjoy expressing it when I choose

My needs come first, before the needs of others

I enjoy being of service to humanity, but do so on my terms

I deserve to heal from this trauma

I am safe healing from this trauma

I release all fear, doubt, guilt and shame around healing from this trauma

How have I been these past four years with regard to this early trauma and its impact?

I have healed completely from it. I connect deeply with myself and with others, enjoying my newfound emotional range. There is such pleasure in discovering the nuances possible in feeling! I serve others only when I choose to, and honour my own needs first. I am no longer gripped with disgust, but walk with my head held high, knowing I am worthy and beautiful. I am fully accepting of who I am in each moment of every day.

Working through all my key traumas over time has proved me right. I am now relaxed and at peace, with no interest in using any addictive substance, like alcohol or sugar. If offered a glass of wine or a chocolate, I enjoy it without needing more.

In fact I'd like to share an interesting story about a client of mine who had an early childhood experience of trauma very similar to mine. The similarities are stark. After her QEC session two days ago, she wrote to me to share how she's been feeling:

> *I am a bit all over the place emotionally (from bliss to tears in 10 seconds kind-of-thing) which although it is a bit unnerving, is essentially all good. It feels like some fundamental internal structure that has been holding me together (in an extremely unhealthy way) is unravelling.*
>
> *I can literally feel my body changing. It is almost like I'm meeting myself for the first time. I did a walking meditation early this morning and had the thought: "Oh, I don't have to control or be afraid of my body or my feelings any more." I was so shocked, as I didn't even know that was what I was doing. But again, it explains the endless ill health, eating disorders and irrational fear of people.*
>
> *I do have this desperate urge to be held and comforted and am trying to self-soothe as best I can. I know that this is my 'child', who I have taken into many adult relationships and been so abused again and again, as she has had no boundaries.*

It was a huge layer of the onion that got peeled with my work with you and my relief is beyond words. I can't thank you enough, Melanie. Honestly, you have no idea (or maybe you do) – being labelled as crazy and unstable whilst getting degrees, excellent jobs, running a business, raising a family, etc. and wondering why the inside feels so shit compared to the outside. After years of endless searching for peace, it finally feels obtainable.

[Permission was obtained from the client to use this quote from her email to me.]

Knowing what I know now, having healed this trauma in myself, I advise my clients that after core trauma work there may be a short period of adjustment. The neurons in the brain are being rewired and it takes time for the entire mind-body to reorganise itself into the new.

It is remarkable how quickly this happens. In a matter of days the person emerges, like a butterfly out of a chrysalis, as a new being, with fading recollection of the old. With neuroplasticity, memory of the old self is pruned away as we organically and naturally move to a new way of being in the world.

CHAPTER 19

The secret

That evening in 1957, when my mother informed me in the semi-dark that she had cancer and was to die within a year, is etched deeply on my soul. What made this traumatic news impossible to live with was the injunction to "keep it a secret between us". How do you present a nine-year-old child with a secret that threatens her own survival in this way? I was emotionally imprisoned with a burden of responsibility beyond my years and my jailer had thrown away the key.

Those years of silent suffering, of watchful service, whilst giving up every single thing that might have brought me joy, are years that shaped me irrevocably. Or so it seemed to me until the age of seventy, when I was finally able to heal.

QEC sentences installed in late 2018:

> ** My ANS is in optimal balance and homeostasis
> ** I release all levels of anxiety and shame

I forgive my mother the cruel and heartless request
to live with the secret of her impending death, and
to serve her every whim at every moment

I forgive her for the impact this had on me – losing
connection with friends and family and pushing me
into unbearable loneliness carrying an impossible
burden

I forgive this selfish act of hers which impacted me
severely in every way, educationally, socially and
personally

I forgive her for narcissistically demanding service
to her needs above all else without care for my
needs

I forgive my father and medical family for being
unable to spot this terrible burden that I carried,
and for accepting my sacrifice to the family as
normal

I forgive my mother her complete denial when
confronted by me ten years afterwards, which in
effect left me imprisoned with they key lost

I forgive myself completely and with compassion for
this sacrifice and for every choice I made because
of it

I release all anger, rage, frustration, guilt, shame,
fear, anxiety, sadness, grief, utter hopelessness
and loneliness, related to this trauma

I restore trust in myself to 100% in speaking out in
my own defence

I am 100% safe within myself, regardless of the
  burdens others attempt to impose on me
I celebrate my determination and commitment to
  keep searching, knowing there HAD to be a key
I am free – and I thank myself for finding the key
I deserve to be free
It is safe to finally be free
I release all fear, doubt, guilt and shame around
  being free

It is strange to write so freely about a topic that has, for almost my entire life, been secretively shut away, out of sight. My imprisonment was too confusing and shameful to ever talk about in my years of therapeutic Gestalt. Throughout my life, until fairly recently, whenever I saw photographs of a prisoner, or a person in a straitjacket, I could relate completely.

Living with lies and betrayal from the person you loved and trusted the most – your mother – is one of the most damaging traumas a person can endure. By the time I was in my twenties, I had shut down to my mother completely, and I remained distant when I finally left South Africa to find a new life in another country. She lived out her old age comfortably in a residential home in Johannesburg called Nazareth House, visited regularly by her Johannesburg grandchildren. She did not play any part in the lives of my children, who never got to know her.

She died during lockdown, last year – 2020 – at the age of ninety-two.

CHAPTER 20

Its time to talk about my father

I loved my father. Genuinely. He loved me too, but it came at an exacting price. He was seldom at home. His work, his sporting pursuits and his relationship with his mistress (later to become his second wife) kept him far away from us. When he was with us on special occasions such as birthdays, I remember being filled with excitement and happiness. He was someone who could give us a laugh – but it didn't go deeper than that. Dad wasn't able to be there emotionally for me or my siblings.

Moving into my teen years, I developed a fear of my father because he placed impossible pressure on me to excel. This pressure spanned academic achievement, sport, music, dance and art. If I showed any interest at all in a new activity, such as learning to play tennis, he would push me with lessons, build me a tennis court and boast loudly to the neighbourhood about 'Melanie, the South African Wimbledon tennis champion to be'. It sounds harmless, but it was excruciatingly embarrassing! If I wasn't keen to climb onto the podium of his Next Great

Idea for me, he would tease and humiliate me for 'having no guts', which was deeply shaming.

The consequence of this high pressure and intense fear of failure felt to me like walking a daily tightrope. It led me to rapidly give up and stop altogether every pursuit he controlled. I am saddened at the loss of all the creative talents I would have loved to have fostered. Dad's narcissism led him to use me in order to receive accolades and recognition for himself. It never occurred to him to ask how I felt; my feelings were irrelevant.

My father was born in 1924 and went to a strict boarding school in South Africa. As a father he engaged proudly in a punitive, controlling style of parenting. His oft-repeated threats, like 'spare the rod and spoil the child' remain with me to this day. He smiled when he beat us, believing he was gifting us with a much-needed lesson. Physical abuse meted out in this way created in me an internalised, sadistic punishing streak which has taken much work to transform.

As an emerging young woman going through puberty, I was struggling with my sexual identity. Being a tomboy who loved riding horses and climbing trees, I was a little confused about my gender. My father would openly criticise my body, telling me I was 'too fat to be liked by any man'. From that time onwards I lost the freedom to be me. I covered myself in a towel when I went swimming, afraid to be seen. In my mid teens, my mother offered me her diet pills: she agreed with him, that life simply would not happen for me if I was fat – even though pictures from that time show that I was hardly overweight at all.

Regardless, the die was cast for – almost – the rest of my life. I believed I was fat and ugly. I also believed I should ingest any substance to lose weight. I smoked, and I took diet pills. Self-disgust and negative body image plagued me throughout my life, as did my internalised harsh critic and occasional sadist.

I was unable to share any of this in therapy because of my high levels of toxic shame. I simply could not be seen to be suffering from these problems; I had to hide behind my mask of middle class professionalism and doctoring.

I'm now appalled at how much was missed in talk therapy.

QEC sentences I installed in early 2019:

> ** My ANS is in optimal balance and homeostasis
> ** I release all levels of anxiety and shame
> I forgive my father for being emotionally absent and physically absent for me and my siblings, and for divorcing my mother when I was 9
> I forgive him for being unable to tune to my needs at all and being interested only in his needs which were always paramount in all interactions with me
> I forgive him his old-fashioned harsh punitive parenting, which included physical beatings and sadistic pleasure at my expense
> I forgive him for becoming narcissistically over-invested in my interests, pushing me to impossible heights and intense fear so that I gave up the interest forever

I forgive him his harsh criticism of my body during puberty, moving me into self hate, insecurity and a distorted self image for the rest of my life

I forgive Mother for introducing me to diet pills and encouraging toxic options to deal with my body, instead of healthy ones

I forgive myself for being utterly disempowered by my father on every level and for believing all the rubbish he gave out

I forgive him for frequently using humiliation and shame to control me and to have a laugh at my expense

I forgive myself for giving up on all my wonderful interests and talents and for being so submissive

I release all anger, frustration, guilt, TOXIC SHAME, humiliation, sadness, fear, anxiety, despair, hopelessness, and all levels of helplessness related to this trauma

I restore trust in myself and my body 100% on all levels

I am 100% safe within myself and in my body at all times

I am finally free of all toxic shame, internal sadistic criticism and torment

I am free of regret about the loss of who I really am

I walk free from the grip of narcissistic parents, and I answer to one call only – that of my soul

I am good enough as I am and happy to be who I am
at my very core
I know that who I am is beautiful, acceptable and
fine, without any need to make changes
I release the lifelong fear of being rejected for how
I look and how I perform
I deserve to be free
It is safe to finally be free
I release all fear doubt guilt and shame around being
free

CHAPTER 21

Loss – my most painful adult trauma

Forty-two years ago today, my daughter Toni died. It is time to share with you my QEC healing work on this trauma.

By the time Toni was born in 1979, my eldest son, Simon, was two years old. Being a mother at home for the first time was a huge heart-opening experience for me. I adored Simon and loved every minute with him. I was eager, after a year or so, to try for another child and so, on the 17th of March 1979, our daughter Toni was born by Caesarean section in Chester hospital. I cannot remember ever again feeling the level of pure joy that I had when I held this beautiful baby. I was ecstatic. My life seemed blessed and wonderful, and my maternal feelings were flowing in full force as I welcomed my second child in to the world.

On Day 4, still in the hospital, Toni began vomiting.

As I've described earlier in this book, the time leading up to her death was a living nightmare, trying to convince local doctors that my baby was desperately ill and that it wasn't that I was simply an 'overanxious mum'. I felt her pain at a gut level but couldn't communicate it. On post mortem it did not surprise me to be told that she had gangrene of the gut from end to end. I knew it and felt it.

What was my trauma here, aside from losing my baby? It was that I felt unable to speak out! I felt that I had no voice and that my baby had died as a result. I had been conditioned to be silent, to be guided by authority figures who 'knew best'. And so I said nothing whilst my entire body felt my daughter's pain and knew she was dangerously ill.

When Toni died I vowed I would never again remain silent on behalf of my children. Today I am not silent about far more – in fact in every imaginable situation I speak out, shout out and even scream from the rooftops when needed!

My healing process with QEC, as you will see below, started with forgiveness for the incompetence of the medical people who did not take Toni's condition seriously until too late. But most of all, I had to forgive myself.

QEC sentences I installed in early 2018:

> ** My ANS is in optimal balance and homeostasis
> ** I release all levels of anxiety and shame
> I forgive the incompetence of all medical personnel involved in Toni's death, which could have and should have been avoided
> I forgive myself, absolutely, on all levels, for being unable and too afraid to let doctors know how ill I knew Toni to be

I forgive my parents and my education for teaching
me to be silent and to follow the voice of authority
above all else

I forgive my husband John for being so traumatised
himself that he was unable to connect and support
me in the way I needed

I release all grief and anguish, anger, frustration,
guilt, shame, heartbreak, despair, longing and
loneliness, related to this trauma

I restore trust in myself and in having a voice and
knowing when to use it

I restore safety within myself for using my voice

I am deeply connected, I know and trust my intuition
and I speak as a single voice from my core

I am unafraid to speak my truth

I deserve to heal from this terrible loss, knowing
I am a good mother

I am safe healing from this trauma

I release all fear, doubt, guilt and shame around
healing from this trauma

I have just been for a walk along the Exe River estuary. The day
is quiet and sunny. Butterflies everywhere in the long grass,
boats bobbing at the water's edge. I reflect on the oh-so-brief
visit I had all those years ago from my daughter Toni, and I am
grateful that she came to turn my life around. I have had much
Gestalt therapy over this loss. It helped me to find peace and to
let it go. But in spite of all those therapeutic years, the ability

to ask for help, to speak when I knew something was not right, was never acquired. I did not find my voice through therapy. The cause was far too deep and entangled with trauma.

Now though, having done QEC on the devastating loss of not saving my baby's life by speaking out, I feel very different. I have a deep inner strength and determination to search for truth. I have found my voice, and I use it when I heal; I use it when I teach; and I use it on behalf of those suffering in the world.

CHAPTER 22

Letters to my parents

My journey has been very long. As I sit here reflecting on it, I am aware of a big change in how I feel towards my parents. Having had a lifetime of disconnection from both my mother and my dad – yearning for connection with them as a child, and then deliberately distancing myself from them as an adult – I am now in a new place.

I feel very connected to each of them right now, and if they were alive I would want to visit them and share what I now understand so well. I can feel my heart is filled with love and compassion for each of them.

Perhaps I can communicate better with letters to each of them:

Dear Mother
I understand exactly how lonely and traumatised you were.
I wish I had known back then what I know now! I would have helped you to really heal and live a completely different life.

I want to thank you for holding so accurately to your end of our soul agreement – that of committing me to the prison of silence, while burdening me with the care of your health. I lost my voice and began to single-handedly search for the key to get it back. I searched in medicine, I searched in psychotherapy and I still couldn't find my voice. I remained trapped in a prison of silence.

And then one day it dawned on me – why not create the key myself?

I have done this.

The key that I made is QEC and it has set me free.

Mother, thank you for your part.

Dear Dad

I thank you for providing in my growing years the fun and laughter and good times at the seaside, which helped to balance out the dark hours of suffering at other times. I know it is what kept me sane.

Above all, thank you for teaching me the meaning of commitment to a purpose. It wasn't applied to all those things you wanted me to commit to, but when the time came and I discovered my purpose, I was totally committed.

Dad, thank you for your part.

Since working on my traumas with QEC, the past four years of my life have been remarkable. I am transformed. I feel I am walking around in a different body. I sometimes touch myself in awe and talk to myself, saying 'Gosh, you really are OK, aren't you?'

It's a sense of wonderment, but it's more than that; I have a deep inner connection with myself. I believe I came to this planet seventy-three years ago, went on a very long journey, and now I am able to be who I really am.

I am free, I am happy, I am at peace.

Most of all I am no longer held in the straitjacket of toxic shame. This is why I can finally write my story, and share the intimacy of my healing process.

Printed in Great Britain
by Amazon